THE EVERYTHING FIRST AID BOOK

Dear Reader,

I'm delighted to share my knowledge of first aid in what I hope you will find an enjoyable and easy way to learn and practice. I had a lot of fun putting the pieces together to make it easy for you to be able to identify signs and symptoms of injuries and what to do in order to respond accordingly. Even if you know nothing or next to nothing about anatomy (parts of the body) and physiology (how the body works), I'm confident that after reading this book you will know how to care for common minor injuries and illnesses.

Like most things, taking personal responsibility is a key aspect of first aid. You should always first use safety and prevention methods and be prepared to respond, but you also need to take care of yourself. I hope you enjoy this book and that you stay healthy and safe.

Nadine Saubers, R.N.

The EVERYTHING® Series

These handy, accessible books give you all you need to tackle a difficult project, gain a new hobby, or even brush up on something you learned back in school but have since forgotten. You can read cover to cover or just pick out information from the four useful boxes.

 Alerts: Urgent warnings

 Essentials: Quick, handy tips

 Facts: Important snippets of information

 Questions: Answers to common problems

When you're done reading, you can finally say you know EVERYTHING®!

DIRECTOR OF INNOVATION Paula Munier

EDITORIAL DIRECTOR Laura M. Daly

EXECUTIVE EDITOR, SERIES BOOKS Brielle K. Matson

ASSOCIATE COPY CHIEF Sheila Zwiebel

ACQUISITIONS EDITOR Kerry Smith

DEVELOPMENT EDITOR Brett Palana-Shanahan

PRODUCTION EDITOR Casey Ebert

ILLUSTRATOR Eric Andrews

Visit the entire Everything® series at *www.everything.com*

THE
EVERYTHING®
FIRST AID
BOOK

How to handle:
Falls and breaks
Insect bites and rashes
Cuts and scrapes
Choking
Burns
Poisoning

Nadine Saubers, R.N.
Technical Review by Vincent Iannelli, M.D.

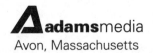

A **adams**media
Avon, Massachusetts

An Everything® Series Book.
Everything® and everything.com® are registered
trademarks of F+W Publications, Inc.

Published by Adams Media, an F+W Publications Company
57 Littlefield Street, Avon, MA 02322 U.S.A.
www.adamsmedia.com

ISBN 10: 1-59869-505-3
ISBN 13: 978-1-59869-505-2

Printed in Canada.

J I H G F E D C B A

Library of Congress Cataloging-in-Publication Data
is available from the publisher.

This publication is designed to provide accurate and authoritative information with regard to the subject matter covered. It is sold with the understanding that the publisher is not engaged in rendering legal, accounting, or other
professional advice. If legal advice or other expert assistance is required, the
services of a competent professional person should be sought.
—From a *Declaration of Principles* jointly adopted by a Committee of the
American Bar Association and a Committee of Publishers and Associations

Many of the designations used by manufacturers and sellers to distinguish
their products are claimed as trademarks. Where those designations appear
in this book and Adams Media was aware of a trademark claim, the designations have been printed with initial capital letters.

The Everything® First Aid Book is intended as a reference volume only, not as
a medical manual. In light of the complex, individual, and specific nature of
health problems, this book is not intended to replace professional medical
advice. The ideas, procedures, and suggestions in this book are intended
to supplement, not replace, the advice of a trained medical professional.
Consult your physician before adopting the suggestions in this book, as well
as about any condition that may require diagnosis or medical attention. The
author and publisher disclaim any liability arising directly or indirectly from
the use of this book.

This book is available at quantity discounts for bulk purchases.
For information, please call 1-800-289-0963.

Visit the entire Everything® series at *www.everything.com*

Acknowledgments

I'm deeply thankful to John Davis and Nancy Deville for their support, which made so many things possible.

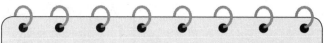

The Top Ten Steps in Emergency Response

1. Call 911 or shout for help until you know someone has heard and called 911, or go for help (either you or someone else needs to call 911).

2. Assess the situation, make sure it's safe before you proceed, and stay calm.

3. Check ABCs, and don't move a person unless there is a life-or-death reason to do so. Ask the injured person what happened.

4. If a person is choking or can't breathe and you are trained in CPR, do the Heimlich maneuver and begin rescue breathing. If the person doesn't have a pulse, start CPR.

5. For any bleeding, apply direct, even pressure.

6. Manage for shock if the person is chilled, short of breath, nauseous, clammy, and pale.

7. Look for a Medic Alert bracelet, necklace, or identification tag (or ID card or driver's license) for any medical history or special needs.

8. After you have stabilized the injured person, go get professional medical help.

9. Don't give the ill or injured person anything to eat or drink, including medications.

10. Wait for the ambulance to arrive while comforting the ill or injured person.

First-Aid Myths

This book's intention is to give you solid first-aid principles and an introduction to emergency response. The most important first step in first aid is to do no further harm. The correct principles for action are covered in detail in the book, but the following list briefly outlines some of the more common first-aid myths.

- Never slap a choking person on the back—let the person cough and the object may dislodge itself. If the person stops coughing or breathing, then perform the Heimlich maneuver.
- Never cut and suck the skin of or apply a tourniquet to a person with a snakebite. Sucking may introduce more bacteria and spread the venom, and a tourniquet will cut off blood supply to the area.
- Peeing on a jellyfish sting won't help the pain.
- Don't breathe into a paper bag for hyperventilation.
- Don't drink alcohol to warm up when cold, it will only lead to hypothermia in cold weather.
- Don't drink alcohol for a toothache or any other pain.
- Don't put butter, Crisco, or any other type of grease on a burn; grease can trap heat and lead to infection and scarring.

- Don't put a raw steak on a black eye or any other injury; the bacteria on the meat may contaminate the wound or the eye.
- Don't use hydrogen peroxide to clean wounds, it may kill the body's defensive cells that are rushing to the wound to take care of invading bacteria.
- People don't swallow their tongues during seizures, so don't try to hold the tongue or put anything in the mouth. Don't restrain the person either.
- Don't squeeze the stinger on a bee sting or try to pull it out with tweezers—this will squeeze venom into the wound; use a credit card to scrape it away.
- Don't throw your head back during a nosebleed—it will cause blood to run down your throat and you may vomit. Instead, lean forward slightly and pinch your nose for ten full minutes.
- If you have something embedded in your skin, you should not pull it out if there is a chance the object is sealing a wound and preventing bleeding. Get medical help if you are not sure.
- Don't continue to run with shin splints; running while injured will increase your injury.
- Don't put vinegar on a sunburn; instead, apply cool compresses.
- You can't stop motion sickness by staring at a point on the horizon.
- Poison ivy is not contagious, but the oil is. If the oil is on you, it can be spread to others.
- Don't use rubbing alcohol to cool down a fever—it will absorb into the skin and may cause further illness.

Contents

Introduction

Every day when you take care of a worrisome symptom, tend to a child's wound, or administer emergency care, you are practicing first aid. This manual contains simple instructions and in some cases life-saving health-care techniques for you to study and refer to in order to take care of the most common nonserious illnesses and injuries. You'll also learn how to identify signs and symptoms and how to understand the difference between a minor injury or illness and those that are more serious. When things do get serious, you'll know how to respond so that you can help others until they can get professional medical care. Knowing what steps to take to prevent illness and injury prevention are just as important for your health and safety as caring for the resulting injury or illness; in fact, prevention should be your first step. That's why this manual is packed with tips and suggestions to keep your home, work, and vacations safe.

Emergencies large and small happen fast and there may not be any time to read instructions, so review some of the basic procedures in this book ahead of time. Every section is designed to give you an overview of what symptoms to look for, how to treat symptoms of illness or injury, when to call 911 for life-threatening emergencies, and when to see your doctor or go to an emergency department. And for emergencies that require basic life-support measures, you are always directed to Chapter 2 so that you can identify what may be happening, including signs of a heart attack, an introduction to CPR, using an automated defibrillator, what to do for a choking person, and how to deal with shock. Follow the instructions in this manual carefully and call for help when you need to.

Many people feel uncomfortable or foolish seeking help, particularly calling 911. That is why signs and symptoms are clearly outlined in each section, as well as when it is absolutely necessary to call for help. Although this manual is intended to be a complete guide, it is not intended to take the place of professional medical advice. Nor should it be used to diagnose and treat illnesses and injuries or to develop a treatment plan for any health problem without consulting your doctor or other qualified medical provider. Nothing takes the place of formal training with hands-on experience, so along with reading and using this manual, you should get certified in basic life support (CPR) and take a formal first-aid class.

Remember, take good care of yourself and of your family, see your doctor for regular checkups, and be prepared for anything in between.

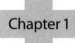

First-Aid Basics

First aid is complex and situation specific, so the more informed and better trained you are the more prepared you are to deal with any unexpected illness or injury. When someone suffers an injury or sudden illness, first aid is your initial course of action. But first aid is more than having a properly stocked first-aid kid; it is being able to prevent, prepare for, recognize, and easily take care of small accidents, and knowing what to do in the case of an emergency. You can treat most common illnesses and injuries when you know what to do, but first you must decide if first aid will be adequate or if you need professional help. And when the condition warrants measures beyond first aid, knowing how to act until help arrives can save someone's life.

Don't Panic!

Being prepared is the best way to avoid panic. Being ready for anything will help you to stay calm, sum up the situation quickly, and proceed with more efficient, capable action. Being prepared will ensure you are composed and self-assured, which will help calm the injured party.

In order to be prepared, make sure to post emergency telephone numbers near the phones in your home and office. Important numbers to keep in addition to 911 are the fire department, the nearest hospital, the Poison Control Center (1-800-222-1222), and your family doctor. Encourage family members with serious medical conditions to wear a Medic Alert tag or bracelet, and keep a list of your family members' medical conditions along with your emergency numbers. Also, have an escape plan from your home and practice it with your children. Keep a fire extinguisher on hand and show all your family members how to use it.

 Fact

You can obtain Medic Alert identification at your pharmacy or doctor's office. These jewelry identification tags are usually engraved with your primary medical conditions (e.g., allergies), ID number, and twenty-four-hour emergency-response-center number.

The Proper Supplies

In order to properly administer first aid, you will need a good first-aid kit. The better stocked and organized your first-aid kit is, the more likely you are to effectively respond to emergencies in your home. Keep a written list of kit supplies in your home, along with your emergency plan, and be sure to restock the kit as needed and replace items with expired dates, items that have been used, or anything with an open package or broken seal that is supposed to be sterile. Keep a first-aid manual like this one with your kit, along with your list of emergency phone numbers, your list or chart of family's medical conditions and medications, and a flashlight.

Be sure to keep first-aid supplies out of the reach of children and pets, as many first-aid supplies are potentially hazardous. Your kit should be in an accessible place, but not one that a child or pet could easily reach, either on their own or with the help of a chair, for instance.

The Right Container

Use a container with a strong handle that can be closed securely, and clearly mark it "First-Aid Kit." Commercial kits can be purchased from many sources, but any large, well-built plastic fishing-tackle box or toolbox works great, and is usually much cheaper.

Ideally, you want your kit to be light enough to carry, but large enough to hold all necessary items in an organized and easily accessible format. It should be dust proof, waterproof, and sturdy enough to resist damage from falling or crushing.

The Right Location

Store your kit safely in a cool, dry location inside your home. Avoid storing it in the garage or laundry room because of the potential harm to its contents from moisture and temperature extremes. Pick a location in your home that is central and accessible to everyone who will be using the kit.

The Right Contents

The ideal kit that will prepare you for most injuries and household emergencies should include the following items:

- Benadryl (generic Diphenhydramine)
- Antibiotic ointment or cream
- Activated charcoal (only use if instructed by the Poison Control Center)
- Antacid (liquid)
- Calamine lotion
- Antihistamine cream
- 1% hydrocortisone cream
- Povidone-iodine solution
- Aspirin, acetaminophen, and ibuprofen
- Sterile eye-wash solution
- Epinephrine auto-injector kit (if prescribed by your doctor)
- Extra prescribed medications (such as inhalers)

Your kit should also contain bandages and dressing supplies including:

- Commercial Band-Aid bandages
- Sterile cotton balls
- Cotton-tipped swabs
- Sterile gauze (pads and rolls)

- Elastic bandage rolls
- Extra bandage clips
- Butterfly bandages
- Sterile eye patches
- Regular adhesive bandages (multiple sizes)
- Adhesive tape (waterproof and stretchable)
- Triangular bandages
- Large foil-lined bandage

Fact

Epinephrine is for emergency use on persons with sudden, severe symptoms or reactions to any allergen such as certain foods, insect stings, and inhaled allergens. If anyone in your family has ever had such a reaction, ask your family doctor to prescribe an Epinephrine auto-injector and to instruct you on how to use it.

Additionally you should include tools and other items such as:

- Bulb syringe
- Medicine spoon (transparent tube marked with typical dosage amounts)
- Small paper cups
- Clean cloths and tissues
- Hand sanitizer
- Digital thermometer (and rectal thermometer for babies less than one year old)

- Small jar of petroleum jelly
- Sterile disposable gloves
- Disposable CPR face mask
- Safety pins
- Scissors (the sharp, angular style with rounded end)
- Tweezers
- Tooth-preservation kit
- Space blanket
- Penlight
- Small pad of paper and pencil
- Emergency candle and waterproof matches
- Disposable self-activating cold and hot packs
- Magnifying glass
- Whistle

Alert!

Aspirin and children's aspirin should never be given to children under age sixteen who have flu-like symptoms or chickenpox. Aspirin may cause Reye's syndrome, which is a life-threatening condition affecting the nervous system and liver.

When preparing your kit, think about your family's medical history, such as drug allergies and risk factors, and keep these drug warnings in mind. Aspirin, ibuprofen, and other nonsteroidal anti-inflammatory (NSAID) drugs may cause stomach bleeding and kidney injury even when taken as directed. The risk is generally higher in people older than fifty-nine, those with stomach ulcers, and anyone who takes blood-thinning drugs or steroids while taking NSAID medications for an extended period. Acetaminophen carries a risk of severe liver damage when people take more than the recommended dose or have three or more alcoholic drinks while taking it. Many over-the-counter medicines (OTC) contain acetaminophen, so check the label of all medicines to make sure you are not exceeding the recommended maximum dose of four grams or four thousand milligrams for a healthy adult in a twenty-four-hour period.

 Essential

Your family medical list or chart should include any information needed for reference by you, paramedics, or doctors including shot records with dates, medical problems and conditions, medications, and allergies.

Gathering Medical Information

Your family medical history is a complete record of health information from three generations of relatives that helps doctors recognize the many factors that your family has in common, including genes, environment, and lifestyle. This medical history will give clues to medical conditions that may run in your family, along with certain patterns of disorders, to determine your risk of developing a particular condition such as heart disease, high blood pressure, stroke, certain cancers, and diabetes.

Compile an information record for all family members that includes their full name, birth date, allergies, history of illnesses, current and past medications, immunization records, history of injuries, any disabilities, rehabilitations, addiction and substance-abuse history and treatment, past hospitalizations, and surgeries. Include any contact information that a first responder may need in case of disasters and in case of times where there may not be anyone to provide the necessary information.

Make sure you also record the name and contact information of your doctors, your insurance coverage, who to notify in case of emergency, and even your religious preference in your medical-information record.

Calling 911

You may be afraid, embarrassed, or wary of calling 911 if you are not sure whether the medical condition or complaint is really an emergency.

There are many conditions that require immediate attention, and you should not wait before calling 911. Instead of risking serious consequences or death if you are not sure, it's wise to call for help. The following are conditions that warrant calling 911, although certainly not an exhaustive list:

- Severe allergic reaction
- Chest pain or heart attack, shortness of breath

- Severe asthma attack or respiratory arrest
- Loss of consciousness or responsiveness
- Confusion, dizziness and fainting, or seizures
- Drug overdose, poisoning, or chemical exposure
- Heat stroke
- Rectal bleeding, bloody diarrhea, bleeding with weakness, or vomiting blood
- Blurred speech, weakness, any signs of stroke
- Uncontrolled bleeding, including nosebleeds
- Serious burns
- Broken bones accompanied by signs of shock or spinal injury
- Suicidal behavior, self-harming or violent behavior

 Alert!

If you have warning signs of a heart attack, call 911 immediately—there is a very limited amount of time before damage to the muscle of the heart is permanent. Emergency medical services (EMS) are trained to treat cardiac arrest on scene and in transit, and you will be treated faster at the hospital if you arrive by ambulance.

The dispatcher's computer is likely to show your location, unless you are on a cell phone or calling from work or another location where the phones are connected to a switchboard. Try to remain calm and answer all questions quickly and as accurately as you are able. The dispatcher will need all of the following information.

- Nature of the emergency
- When emergency first occurred
- Exact location or address where help is needed
- Phone number that you are calling from
- Your name and who else is involved

Follow all instructions given by the 911 dispatcher and stay on the phone until the dispatcher tells you to hang up, or for as long as it is safe to do so. Stay calm, be clear, listen to the dispatcher carefully, and answer as concisely as possible.

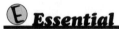 **Essential**

It's the 911 dispatcher's job to know how to ask the right questions. Pay attention and answer all questions as best you can. Don't hang up until you are told to; if you are on a cell phone you may have to give your exact location and other information as your location will not be visible to the dispatcher.

Informing Kids

Teach young children how to phone 911 by using a toy phone or an old, nonworking cell phone. Explain to them that emergencies include car accidents, crimes like when someone is hurting another person or breaking into the house, when someone in the family is suddenly very sick (for example, having a hard time speaking, breathing, or turns blue), if anyone collapses or passes out, or if the house is on fire.

 Fact

> Most children over five years of age are capable of understanding and learning how and when to call 911. Instruct children to call 911 only for real emergencies. Make sure they understand that the police and firefighters will come when they call 911.

Universal Precautions

The threat of communicable disease is a hazard in performing first aid. You should follow some standard precautions (called universal precautions) and use personal protection equipment like gloves, a CPR barrier, or eye protection. Universal precautions protect aid providers from exposure to HIV (the virus that causes AIDS), hepatitis B, and other blood-borne germs when exposed to blood, certain body fluids (including semen and vaginal fluid), and tissue from anyone who is infectious. Universal precautions should also be taken for cerebrospinal (from the lining of the brain and spinal cord), synovial (joint), pleural (lung), peritoneal (abdominal), pericardial (heart), and amniotic (pregnant uterus) fluids. These guidelines don't apply to other body fluids like saliva, urine, sweat, tears, nasal secretions, sputum, and feces unless they contain blood. Professional universal precautions include:

1. Wash your hands before and after any medical intervention.
2. Wear gloves whenever you are in contact with another's blood, body secretions, or tissues even if the person you are helping is a family member.
3. Wear a facemask or body gown whenever there is a possibility of blood splashing onto the rescuer.
4. Dispose of contaminated sharp objects in the appropriate puncture-proof container.
5. Dispose of all contaminated equipment in an appropriate biohazard container.

While you may not have all the equipment necessary, these professional guidelines will steer you in the right direction. As a layperson, you should try and follow these precautions as closely as possible.

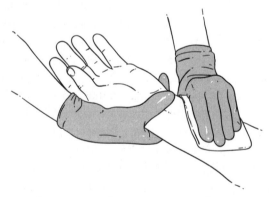

Rescuer using gloves as a protective barrier

Alert!

Practice universal precautions when coming in contact with blood or any body secretions or fluids that may also contain blood to protect your own health and even save lives.

To carry-out universal precautions against infectious disease, you should use a protective barrier when you are providing care to anyone, even if you know the person well. In this day and age, it's just common sense to avoid contact with an unknown potential source of infection. If you don't have gloves, improvise and use something like plastic wrap and wash your hands thoroughly before and after providing any care.

Essential

Universal precautions mean you are to be careful and not take chances; it doesn't mean that you don't provide care!

The Proper Training

While this book is designed to be a comprehensive resource, providing first-aid basics, nothing can replace the hands-on learning you get from formal training in a classroom setting. Anyone can learn first aid, and by learning new lifesaving skills and updating past knowledge, you will feel and act more confident at home and work and while traveling.

Many organizations offer first-aid classes, such as the American Red Cross, the American Heart Association, and the National Safety Association; and other local EMS organizations offer Basic Life Support (BLS) classes. Some occasionally offer free one-day classes to the community; most charge a small fee for a one- to two-day course in CPR and basic first aid.

Chapter 2

Emergency Response

It's well known that in order to save lives, CPR needs to begin immediately after a person collapses or "witnessed arrest" occurs (when someone sees the event occur). But only approximately one-third or less of people respond in witnessed arrest situations, and even when CPR is begun immediately it is often done incorrectly. That's why it's important to become certified in CPR and Automated External Defibrillators (AED) and to take the recommended renewal certification classes. By learning CPR, you can help preserve life, limit disability, restore health, and even reverse clinical death in emergency situations.

History of CPR

The origins of cardiopulmonary resuscitation (CPR) can be traced back to 1740, when the Paris Academy of Sciences first formally recommended mouth-to-mouth resuscitation for near-drowning victims. Over a hundred years later in 1891, the first documented and effective chest compression in humans was performed by Dr. Friedrich Maass. Through the years the use of external chest compressions in human resuscitation was attempted and analyzed, and it was proven that expired air by a rescuer is sufficient to oxygenate an unresponsive person. CPR was then officially developed and instituted in 1960, and a program by the American Heart Association (AHA) provided CPR training and encouraged the use of CPR by the general public. The American Red Cross and other agencies came on board to institute performance standards, standardized training, and certification for CPR for intervention of sudden cardiac arrest and acute life-threatening cardiopulmonary problems.

Every five years the AHA guidelines for CPR and emergency cardiac care are reviewed, improved, and updated to improve survival rates of life-threatening events. AHA establishes these guidelines with the cooperation of other organizations, peer-reviewed studies, and other systematic evidence-based study and review. The following is a review of the most recent (2005) AHA CPR and resuscitation protocol.

The ABCs of First Aid

There are three critical steps in emergency first aid. A person needs all three common denominators to live, and basic life support or CPR, together with early defibrillation, is proven to improve long-term survival after a cardiac arrest. While this book outlines the basic steps for cardiopulmonary resuscitation, it should not be relied on for instruction; rather, it should be used for an introduction and followed by formal training and exercises. You can find CPR and first-aid classes by calling the American Heart Association or the American Red Cross.

The ABCs of first aid is a mnemonic that stands for airway, breathing, and circulation:

- **Airway:** Is the airway unobstructed? Use measures to clear the airway.
- **Breathing:** Is the person breathing? Start rescue breathing.
- **Circulation:** Is the person's heart beating? Start chest compressions.

Basic CPR and AED

According to the AHA, CPR is not a single skill, but a series of assessments and interventions, and cardiac arrest is not just one problem, so the steps of CPR will vary depending on the type or cause of the arrest. For the purposes of this book, only lay-rescuer techniques and methods will be reviewed. It's worthy to note that lay rescuers are no longer taught to check for pulse or signs of circulation or taught to provide rescue breathing without chest compressions for an unresponsive person. Take the following steps when you witness anyone over the age of one year old collapse:

1. Assess that it is safe to approach the fallen person.
2. Use protective equipment and follow universal precautions. If you are able to, use common sense, and stay away from any obvious hazards.
3. Attempt to wake the person by rubbing your knuckles firmly against the sternum (breastbone) and shouting, "Are you okay?"
4. If the person fails to rouse, immediately call 911 or shout for help, depending on your situation. If there is an AED available, also shout for someone to bring it.

5. If the person becomes conscious, is moaning, or moves, do not start CPR.

6. Call 911 if the person is not able to speak or appears confused. If the person does not wake, begin CPR and use an AED if available.

An AED is a small, portable electronic device that is used to deliver an electric shock in an attempt to disrupt or stop abnormal electrical activity in the heart. Abnormal electrical activity correlates with an abnormal heart rhythm, and a continual abnormal rhythm is not sufficient to pump blood and deliver oxygen through the body. An AED shock cannot restart a dead heart; the heart must have a rhythm (even though the rhythm is abnormal). The AED will automatically diagnose any cardiac arrhythmia when attached by leads to an unconscious person. When you see one of these lethal rhythms, you can then treat the person with the AED electrical therapy or a shock (defibrillation) that may interrupt the arrhythmia and allow the heart to re-establish a normal and effective rhythm. You can learn how to use an AED in many first-aid, first-responder, and CPR classes.

ⓔ *Essential*

The AHA recommends that rescuers push hard, push fast (100 compressions per minute), and allow complete chest recoil between compressions, with minimal interruptions in compressions, for all persons.

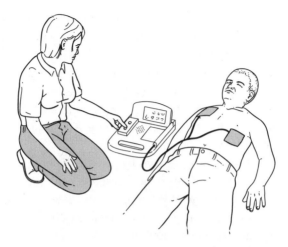

An AED is used to interrupt a lethal heart rhythm

The steps for performing CPR are:

1. Open the airway using the head-tilt, chin-lift method—
   one hand on the forehead, fingers of the other hand
   under the bony part of the lower jaw, near the chin.
   Tilt the head back, gently lift the jaw, making sure
   not to close the mouth or push on soft parts beneath
   the chin. Avoid lifting the neck in the case of spinal
   injury.
2. Check for normal breathing by putting your ear to the
   person's mouth and turning your head to look for chest
   movement, while listening for air flowing through the
   mouth or nose and trying to detect breath on your
   cheek. A person with periodic gasping is most likely
   in cardiac arrest and needs CPR.

3. If there are no signs of breathing, pinch the nose; make a seal over the mouth with yours and give the person a breath strong enough for you to see the chest rise. When the chest falls, repeat the rescue breath once more for a total of two breaths. If available, use a CPR mask as a barrier between your mouth and the person's mouth that you are rescuing. These first three steps are called "rescue breathing."

4. Begin chest compressions by placing the heel of your hand in the middle of the chest, over the lower half of the breastbone at the nipple line. Place your other hand on top and lace your fingers together (heel of one hand on chest, heel of the other hand on top of that hand) and compress the chest about one to two inches. Allow the chest to recoil completely, and then perform thirty compressions, at a rate of 100 compressions per minute.

5. After thirty chest compressions, immediately repeat the two rescue breaths. Open the airway with head-tilt, chin-lift again. This time, go directly to rescue breaths without checking for breathing again. Give one breath, making sure the chest rises and falls, then give another.

6. Perform the cycle of thirty compressions followed by two breaths for about two minutes. Then stop and recheck for breathing. If the person is not breathing, continue chest compressions and rescue breaths.

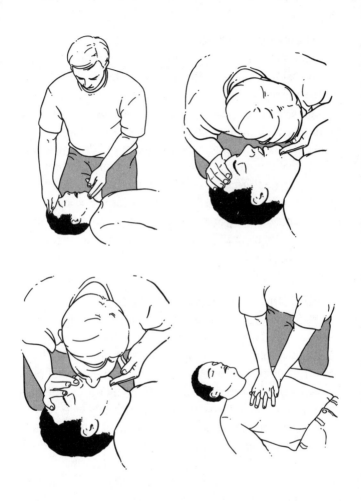

Steps of CPR

Other Considerations

The AHA now recommends that a series of thirty compressions followed by two breaths (compression-ventilation ratio of 30:2) be given to all persons, regardless of age. Continue the cycle of compressions and rescue breathing until professional help arrives or until the person recovers and begins breathing. In children age one to eight, use one or two hands as necessary to compress the chest one-third to one-half the depth of the chest. For the unresponsive infant or child, perform five cycles of thirty compressions and two breaths for about two minutes before leaving the child to call 911 and get an AED if one is available.

CPR for Newborns and Infants

Newborn CPR has different recommendations than those for infants. But the recommendations for newborn CPR only apply to newborns in the first hours after birth until the newborn leaves the hospital, so the general public needs only to be concerned with infant CPR guidelines that apply to babies less than approximately one year of age. The rescue-breathing rate for infants with pulses is about forty to sixty breaths per minute, with chest compression to one-third the depth of the chest. Deliver ninety compressions and thirty ventilations per minute. Compress the infant chest just below the nipple line (on lower half of sternum) using two fingers (rather than a whole hand) to compress the chest with a compression-ventilation ratio of 30:2.

Problems Associated with CPR

Some of the problems the AHA has identified regarding performing CPR are excessive ventilation given during CPR and compressions that are interrupted too frequently and that are often too slow and too shallow. It's believed that bystanders may be reluctant to perform CPR because it seems too complicated and difficult to remember. That's why in recent updates the AHA has made attempts to simplify the steps by making the compression-ventilation ratio used the same for infants, children, and adults. The same update has been issued for chest compressions in children and adults.

While it's been surmised that the public is afraid of contracting diseases and is therefore reluctant to perform mouth-to-mouth resuscitation, the data illustrates that transmission of infection is very low; nonetheless, use of a barrier device (CPR mask) while giving ventilations is still encouraged. If you are still reluctant to give mouth-to-mouth ventilations, at least call for help and start chest compressions immediately.

Alert!

If you or a family member have a preexisting heart condition or are at high risk for heart failure, your doctor may be able to prescribe an AED that's at least partially covered by your medical plan.

Recovery Position

The recovery position is a technique used in first aid for all unconscious people who are breathing. This includes anyone over the age of one year old who has started breathing after being given CPR, those who may be unconscious or nearly unconscious but are still breathing, those who are too inebriated to assure their continued breathing, persons of near drowning, and in cases of suspected poisoning.

An unconscious person who is lying face up is in a position that may result in obstruction to the airway. When a person is laying face up, the tongue may relax to the back of the throat and fluids such as blood or vomit can pool in the back of the throat and obstruct the airway. Also, in the face-up position, the esophagus is tilting down slightly from the stomach toward the throat, and when combined with loss of muscular control that occurs when someone is unconscious, this can lead to what is called passive regurgitation—when the stomach contents flow up into the throat. Aside from airway obstruction, any fluid collecting in the back of the throat can flow down into the lungs and the acid from the stomach that is in that fluid can damage the lungs, a condition known as aspiration pneumonia. In many instances, the actual injury or illness that caused unconsciousness will not be fatal, but the resulting passive regurgitation or aspiration pneumonia will be.

A very common cause of death is excessive consumption of alcohol that leads to unconsciousness followed by all or some of these events. While in the recovery position, the force of gravity keeps the tongue from obstructing the airway and prevents fluids from flowing the wrong way. This, coupled with raising the chest above the ground, protects the person while aiding breathing.

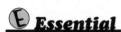

Essential

You must suspect spinal injury and use measures to stabilize the neck if the person is unconscious because of an accidental fall, collision, or any other trauma.

As in all first-aid situations, assess the area for safety before approaching the unconscious person. Next, assess the person for the ABCs. If there is no need to perform CPR or if you already have performed CPR and the person begins breathing, then put the person into the recovery position. If there is no suspicion of spinal or neck injury, you want to place the person into what is called the lateral recovery position:

1. With the person lying on his back with legs straight out, kneel on one side, facing him. Position the person's arm that is closest to you perpendicular to his body, with his elbow flexed. Then position the other arm across the body, resting the hand across the torso.
2. Bend the leg that is farthest from you up; the knee elevated, reach behind the knee and pull the thigh toward you.

3. Use your other arm to pull the shoulder farthest from you while rolling the body toward you. Maintain the upper leg in a flexed position so that the body is stabilized.

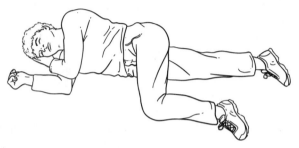

Lateral recovery position

Because people who stay in this position for an extended period of time may experience nerve compression, you may move the person from side to side every thirty minutes if emergency rescue is taking a long time to arrive. In case of spinal injury, any other movement of the unstabilized neck will carry a risk of causing permanent paralysis or other injuries, so movement should be minimized. The only reason to move a person with a suspected spinal injury into a recovery position is if you must drain vomit from the airway. And then you should use what is called HAINES modified recovery position (High Arm IN Endangered Spine). In this modified position, raise one of the injured person's arms above the head (in full abduction) while turning the person's body in order to support the head and neck for less neck movement.

In a suspected spinal or neck injury, your first priority is keeping the airway open, so if the person is breathing, leave them in the position you found them. But if breathing stops, regardless of potential for increased injury to the person, you must continue ABCs: airway, breathing, and circulation. Breathing is the first priority; everything else is second.

An unconscious pregnant woman should always be positioned in the recovery position on her left side, and anyone with wounds to the torso should be placed with the wounds closest to the ground to decrease any chance of blood pooling in the lungs.

Place a baby less than a year old in a modified recovery position by holding the infant in your arms, head tilted downward, in order to prevent the tongue from obstructing the airway or the infant from inhaling vomit. In all cases, continue to monitor the person's level of response, pulse, and breathing until help arrives.

Signs of Heart Attack

Sometimes heart attacks are sudden and there is no doubt what is happening, but those are the minority. Most heart attacks begin slowly with very mild discomfort and pain. The biggest mistake is when people aren't sure and they wait too long to seek help. If you or anyone you know has the following symptoms, seek help immediately:

- Chest discomfort such as uncomfortable pressure, squeezing, fullness, or pain in the center of the chest lasting more than a few minutes, or that comes and goes

- Discomfort in other areas of the upper body including pain or discomfort in one or both arms, the back, neck, jaw, or stomach
- Shortness of breath
- A cold sweat, nausea, or lightheadedness

Women are more likely to have some of the other common symptoms, in particular back or jaw pain, shortness of breath, nausea, and vomiting. Even if you are not sure, it's wise to call 911. If you are not able to access Emergency Medical Services (EMS), have someone else drive you to the hospital immediately. Never drive yourself unless there is no other option.

 Question?

Are the symptoms of a heart attack the same for both men and women?
Women have the same symptoms as men but, are more prone to also have back or jaw pain, shortness of breath, nausea, and vomiting. You need to seek immediate medical help for any symptoms, not just the "classic" symptoms of a heart attack.

What Is Happening?
The heart functions both mechanically and electrically. It pumps blood by contracting, which you are able to feel as a pulse—the mechanical function. The heart

also has cells that regulate the mechanical system by transmitting electrical signals through conduction pathways, stimulating the muscle tissue to contract—the electrical function. The rate of electrical stimulation or pulses normally correlates with the rate of heart-muscle contractions or beats, and should be between sixty and eighty times per minute at rest, increasing with exertion.

The pumping chambers of the heart are the ventricles. If they suddenly stop effectively contracting and pumping blood into the body, Sudden Cardiac Arrest (SCA) occurs. The heart then has a disorganized and abnormal rhythm and spasmodic twitching called "ventricular fibrillation" (VF) that is ineffective in pumping blood to the body. The person in VF or V fib usually has no pulse because the heart is not pumping blood, and they will then become unresponsive, stop breathing, and die within minutes without intervention.

Choking

Choking occurs when an object gets stuck in the throat and partly or completely blocks the airway. Signs of choking include:

- Pointing to throat, hands crossed on throat (universal sign of choking)
- Gasping or coughing
- Signs of panic
- Difficulty speaking
- Red face that steadily turns blue
- Loss of consciousness

Alert!

Never slap any person on the back you think might be choking. A baby who is crying, has a strong cough, and appears to be breathing well should be placed in a sitting position and allowed to finish coughing. Never stick your fingers down a baby's throat, or anyone else's, in an attempt to remove an object while they are coughing.

When you suspect someone is choking, ask her, "Are you choking?" If the person is able to answer you, don't do anything because it's likely that she will free the food or object on her own. In the case of actual choking, the person will not be able to talk and you need to help them. Call 911 if the person can't talk, make noise, or breathe well or is unconscious, then perform the Heimlich maneuver as outlined below. If the person is unconscious, lay her on her back. Check the person's mouth for any visible obstruction and try to dislodge it using a finger sweep. If you are unable to do so, begin mouth-to-mouth resuscitation and CPR. Continue to check inside the person's mouth for any signs of the foreign body as the chest compressions of CPR may dislodge it.

Heimlich Maneuver

The Heimlich maneuver (pronounced Hi-mlick) is a technique whereby you administer abdominal thrusts to yourself or to a person who is choking. The Heimlich maneuver is recommended for use in clearing a blocked airway in conscious adults and children over the age of one; it is not meant to be used for choking infants under age one. The act of abdominal thrust lifts the diaphragm and forces air from the lungs, similar to a coughing action, so that the foreign body in an airway may be moved and expelled.

The steps to perform the Heimlich maneuver on a choking person are:

1. Stand behind the person, wrap your arms around the waist, and tip the person slightly forward.
2. Make a fist with one hand and place it slightly above the navel.
3. Grasp your fist with your other hand and press forcefully into the abdomen with quick, upward thrusts, using force as if you were attempting to lift the person up.
4. Continue the thrusts until the foreign body is dislodged.

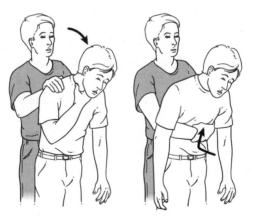

Heimlich maneuver

The steps to perform the Heimlich maneuver on yourself if you are choking are:

1. Place your fist just slightly above your navel.
2. Grasp your fist with your other hand, bend over a hard surface like a chair or countertop, and thrust your fist inward and upward.

To clear an airway obstruction of a pregnant woman or obese person, place your fists closer to the chest, right above the joining of the ribs at the base of the breastbone, and follow the Heimlich maneuver steps. When a choking person is unconscious, lower the person on her back onto the floor. Clear the airway using the head-tilt method. If you can see the blockage, reach a finger into the mouth and sweep it out (finger sweep), using caution not to push the object deeper into the airway. If you are unable to remove the obstructing object and the person doesn't respond, you must begin CPR. In this case, there is a chance that the chest compressions used in CPR will free the object so recheck the mouth at regular intervals.

In the case of a choking infant younger than age one, sit with the infant face down on your forearm, positioned securely on your thigh. Thump the infant firmly and gently five times with the heel of your hand in the middle of the back. The back blows and the gravity will most likely free the obstruction. If it doesn't work, turn the infant face up on your forearm, head lower than body, and use two fingers positioned over the center of the breastbone just below the nipples and give five quick chest compressions. Continue to repeat the back blows and chest thrusts and if the infant doesn't start breathing, call 911. If you have cleared the obstruction and the infant doesn't start breathing, begin infant CPR. In babies older than age one, only give abdominal thrusts.

 Fact

Unintentional injuries from events such as motor-vehicle crashes, chokings and suffocations, near drownings, bicycle-related crashes, falls, and poisonings are the leading causes of death for children ages fourteen and under. By learning CPR and first aid you could save a child's life!

Swallowing Foreign Objects

Children and adults that have altered states due to illness such as stroke and alcohol abuse, and denture wearers, are more prone than others to accidentally swallowing small foreign objects. Small and hazardous items need to be kept out of children's reach, particularly coins and batteries, both of which are common in households and are frequently swallowed foreign objects. Denture wearers lack the tactile sensation in their mouths that helps prevent inadvertently swallowing items like bones, and need to be especially careful. Foreign objects may get stuck in the esophagus (swallowing passage) and cause symptoms of drooling and retching, pain in the chest area, choking, and difficulty swallowing. After several hours, other symptoms may develop such as vomiting, nausea, stomach pain, blood in the stool, and fever.

First Aid for Swallowing a Foreign Object

For anyone who is experiencing signs of a blocked airway, perform the Heimlich maneuver as outlined for choking. For other persistent symptoms seek medical attention, because in 20 percent of cases the object needs to be removed by your doctor with an endoscope procedure. Any child suspected of swallowing a battery needs to be taken to the emergency department immediately because batteries corrode and release chemicals that can cause severe damage. Other noncaustic items, after the initial discomfort subsides, will often pass through on their own. For any questions or concerns, always consult with your medical-care professional.

Managing Shock

Preventing and managing shock is a matter of life and death in emergencies. When the circulatory system stops working to deliver blood to the body, shock occurs. If the heart beats irregularly, if blood vessels become too dilated, or if a person is losing too much blood, shock may occur. The symptoms of shock are a weak and rapid pulse; disorientation; dizziness or confusion; cold, clammy skin and hands and pale skin; extreme thirst; nausea and vomiting; high level of anxiety; and fingernails that do not blanch with applied pressure (turn white when pressed and color does not return within two seconds).

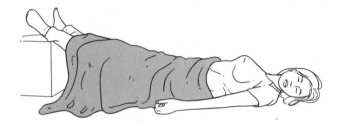

If someone is in shock, elevate her legs, keep her warm, and turn her head to one side if neck injury is not suspected

In emergency situations you must guard the person against shock. Call 911 for help immediately, because you cannot manage shock alone for long, and the person is likely to go into cardiac arrest. Check the ABCs continually while waiting for help and begin CPR if needed. If the head, neck, back, hips, or legs are not injured, lay the person on the ground facing up and elevate the legs to keep critical blood flow to vital organs. Use a towel, a sanitary napkin, or a piece of clothing to apply pressure to open wounds to slow bleeding. Keep the person calm, comfortable, and warm, but never give the person water, even if they claim to be very thirsty. Monitor the person for consciousness and ABCs continually until help arrives.

Chapter 3

Preventive Measures

Most common injuries and sudden illnesses occur in the home, and accidents are the leading cause of death among children and injuries in adults. Human error has been found to be the major cause behind most accidents; that's why preventive measures are so important. This chapter will help keep you and your family safer in the home, with an overview of prevention measures you should take.

An Ounce of Prevention

The proverb, "An ounce of prevention is worth a pound of cure" still holds true; it's so much easier to spend a little time forestalling disasters than it is to deal with them. Take a look at your home, assess any safety issues and unsafe habits, and determine potential hazards. Think about what you can do to correct those danger areas, and take necessary safety and prevention measures.

Toxins

Some products may harm the skin and gain entry through damaged skin. Others are absorbed even if they don't do any skin damage, so wearing protective gloves and clothing is important when working with potentially hazardous products and anything that has a warning label. Many chemical products are particularly damaging to the eyes and require protective goggles (even if you wear glasses) during use. You can buy goggles at many drugstores and home stores.

Alert!

The word "nontoxic" only indicates that a substance may cause little to no adverse reactions if you eat it or inhale it. It does not guarantee that the product is harmless. For illness and allergic reactions, consider that the source may be any product you've used that contains chemicals.

Reading labels and directions will help you determine if it is a product you really want in your home and will instruct you how to use it and what to do in case of emergency ingestion or contact with eyes. Try to avoid products labeled with the words "Caution," "Poison," "Danger," or "Warning."

Anything circulating in the air will enter the bloodstream via your lungs, so good ventilation is essential, along with the use of fans and open windows when using any sort of aerosol or volatile toxin. If you can smell it, then your ventilation is not adequate. Some toxic products don't have odors, so it's a good idea to wear a mask for your own protection.

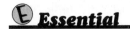
Essential

Remember to never mix products unless the manufacturer's directions say that it's safe to do so. Mixing products may cause toxic or explosive chemical reactions.

After you read the directions, follow them! Keep all lids tightly closed and follow the manufacturer's storage recommendations. If you are able to, work outdoors or take ample fresh-air breaks. Take a break, go outside, or even stop working altogether if you become dizzy, nauseated, or develop a headache.

For pests, baits and traps are the safest pesticides because they do not cause the entire area that you are treating to become toxic, and are designed so that the pest enters the container containing the pesticide and then takes it back to the colony or nest.

Alternatives to insecticides are diatomaceous earth (don't use the swimming-pool variety), B.T. (a microbial insecticide), insecticidal soaps, beneficial nematodes (good bugs that clean up the pesty ones), neem oil (a natural insecticide), and frequent vacuuming. For pet flea control, try alternatives such as enzyme shampoos and using a 50:50 mixture of white vinegar and water sprayed on the pet, weekly washing of pet bedding, and frequent vacuuming.

Store products in their original container with the original label attached, and store flammable products away from corrosive products. After using rags with any flammable products, such as furniture stripper or paint remover, store them in a sealed and labeled, preferably metal, container away from heat or sparks that could ignite them.

Fact

If you are pregnant, try to avoid toxic chemical exposure, because many toxic products have either never been tested for potential harmful effects to an unborn fetus or have been manufactured, sold, and then later found to be toxic and taken off the market.

Fire Safety

The U.S. Fire Administration recommends having working smoke detectors installed in all bedrooms, in rooms outside the bedroom areas, and at least one detector on each story of your house. They also recommend that you test your smoke detectors monthly, replace the batteries once a year, and replace the detectors after ten years of use. Because fires commonly travel along the stairway, you should have escape ladders to help you get out of the second story of a house and practice using them when you practice your escape plan. Never try to put an out-of-control fire out, just leave quickly and call for help. But do keep an ABC or ABCD fire extinguisher in the kitchen, garage, and/or workshop and know how to use it for small, manageable fires.

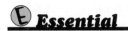
Smoke detectors will give you the chance to escape a fire situation, but you also need to prepare and practice your emergency-exit plan with two ways out from each room. Also be sure to plan a location where the family will meet together outside after escaping.

Keep fireplaces screened and cleaned. Chimneys and stovepipes should be professionally cleaned yearly for creosote, a substance that can ignite and cause a house fire.

Kitchen Safety

The most common kitchen fire is the dry-cooking fire, where the liquid or substance in a pot cooks out and what is left begins to smoke. Grease fires happen when something oily ignites while cooking, causing open flames that can become a disastrous fire. Take the following steps to prevent or control kitchen fires:

- Turn off the stove if you are able to.
- If a pan is on fire and you are able to cover it with a lid, do so.
- Don't ever try to splash water on a grease fire or carry a burning pan outside or to the sink.
- Keep a fire blanket in your kitchen so that you can cover your hands with it and throw it gently over a fire.

- Use timers to remind you of food cooking, even if you think you will remember.
- Keep all flammable items like dish towels and bags away from the stove top.
- Always use potholders or oven mitts, and never dish towels, to handle your hot pots, pans, and baking trays.

 Fact

Electrical outlets that are close to water sources in the kitchen, bathroom, and garage should be protected by Ground-Fault Circuit Interrupters (GFCIs). GFCIs monitor the flow of electricity and automatically cut off the flow of electricity with any variation in the current, thus preventing injury.

Childproofing Your Home

When you have a baby, you should immerse yourself in classes and books on how to protect the baby in your home. The following guidelines will give you an overview on childproofing your home.

Physical Dangers

Electrical outlets tend to fascinate children. Many are down at eye level and they have small inviting holes for curious fingers, thus causing many injuries and even deaths every year by electrocution. Plastic outlet covers and plugs will prevent injuries, and ideally, childproof receptacles can also be installed in place of ordinary outlets.

If you have upper-story windows, you need to install safety bars on them that are childproof but simple for adults to open in case of fire or other emergencies. At the very least, keep windows closed and locked when children are present and never leave small children unattended around open windows. Don't place furniture near windows, potentially allowing children to climb onto sills, and never assume that a screen will protect a child from falling out of any window. Most houses have many items, including furniture, that have a potential to topple, injure, and even cause fatal injuries when pulled or climbed on. You can purchase anti-tip devices for items such as dressers, bookcases, entertainment centers, TVs, appliances, and tall floor lamps. Appliance locks are inexpensive and easy to install and keep doors to ovens and refrigerators safely locked to help protect your child from accidents.

Alert!

The American Academy of Pediatrics discourages the use of mobile baby walkers because they result in thousands of head injuries to babies every year. Today these unsafe, wheel-driven baby walkers are not as readily available, and most experts strongly discourage their use—so politely decline one, even as a hand-me-down.

Make sure to buy a crib that meets federal safety standards and keep the crib mattress tidy. To avoid Sudden Infant Death Syndrome (SIDS), never place an infant face down on any sort of plastic-covered mattress or table. Always keep your crib side-rails up, and strap children securely in anything that has a safety belt, such as a high chair, stroller, or changing table. In order to prevent falls, don't ever leave your baby lying on a bed or couch or changing table; instead, pick the baby up if you need to answer the phone or the door or you forgot something.

When you have babies and toddlers in the house, all of your coffee tables, furniture, and countertops with sharp edges should have protective padding or other specially designed covers attached to the corners. Install hardware-mounted safety gates at the top of every stairway and in between doors that you want to secure. Avoid using pressure-mounted gates because they are not secure enough, and do not use accordion gates because they can trap a child's head.

 Fact

Balloons should never be given to children under eight years old. Always supervise children of any age around balloons; they are easily popped, and if inhaled, small pieces can block the airway. Balloons are not visible on X-rays, so if a child has aspirated a piece of balloon the reason for distress may not be apparent.

Thin plastics are suffocation hazards around babies and children and should be disposed of promptly after tying them in knots. Keep all of your plastic garbage bags and other plastic bags including sandwich bags out of the reach of children. Take the following steps for choking and strangulation prevention:

- Don't give foods such as nuts of any type, hard candy, fruit with seeds, grapes, raw carrots, raw peas, raw celery, cherries with pits, or popcorn to children under age four.
- Avoid garments with drawstrings for small children and babies; cut drawstrings out of hoods, jackets, and waist bands, and cut the strings off of mittens or other items (mobiles and crib toys).
- When your baby has outgrown the stage of just lying and looking at the mobile, take it down and store it securely.
- Tie up window-blind cords out of reach, or use specially designed cord clips.
- Be careful with necklaces and headbands on babies and anything that has the potential to wrap around a baby's neck, such as long telephone cords, pacifiers tied around the neck, and hanging purses or diaper bags.
- Never place your baby face down on soft surfaces such as waterbeds, sheepskin rugs, quilts, mattress covers, soft pillows, beanbags or bead-filled pillows, or near large stuffed animals.

Set the thermostat on your home hot-water heater to 120°F or lower. If you live in an apartment and you are not able to control the water temperature, you should install an anti-scald device that causes the water to slow to a trickle if it reaches a dangerous temperature.

Drowning is a leading cause of death in children under five. All pools and Jacuzzis need to have layers of protection including a pool fence with a self-closing, self-latching gate that prevents access to the water; pool alarms; and close adult supervision when children are present. Child flotation devices are never a replacement for adult supervision. Dump out all water from a wading pool when kids are finished playing every single time you use it. In fact, never leave any body of water sitting around, including pails of water or any other liquid, because toddlers can drown in a matter of minutes in unattended buckets. Babies should never be left unattended in a bath or wading pool even for a second for you to answer the door or phone. Pick up the baby and take him with you! Always stay in the bathroom when you are filling a tub with water.

Firearms need to be stored securely in a locked case, out of the reach of children. They must be stored unloaded and uncocked, and padlocks that prevent the cylinder from locking into place should be attached to all revolvers. Teach and emphasize to your children that guns are not toys and should never be touched or played with.

Children and Toxic Dangers

Every year thousands of children go to emergency rooms due to accidental poisoning. There are many safety latches and locks for cabinets and drawers on the market today that are designed to keep out tiny hands and that you can buy at any home store or general retail outlet.

According to EPA guidelines, all homes built before 1978 that are being remodeled should be tested for lead paint. Any baby items, furniture, or toys that were made before 1978 may have a finish or paint that contains dangerously high levels of lead.

Medicines, including over-the-counter medicine and vitamins, are all potentially hazardous household products. Never try to get your children to take a vitamin or medication by calling it candy.

 Fact

The most common cause of death by poisoning in children comes from accidental overdoses from the iron in children's vitamins. Keep all medications in a single locked location and call the Poison Control Center immediately for any suspected ingestion of vitamins by children.

Keep all medications, vitamins, supplements, and over-the-counter medication securely locked away, never sitting on a counter. Even if a label states it is child resistant that does not guarantee it is childproof. Make sure that grandparents and all other child caretakers understand the potential hazards of medications and vitamins and the necessary safety measures, because 20 percent of accidental poisonings of children happen when they are in the care of their grandparents.

Protecting the Elderly

Older persons often lack strength and flexibility and may have bones that tend to be porous and more brittle. Further, their senses of sight, hearing, touch, and smell are likely to decline with less accurate judgment and reaction time. All of these factors make the elderly more vulnerable to accidents. The elderly need to take precautions including the following basics:

- Post emergency numbers next to each telephone and have several cordless phones available if possible.
- Install door lever-action handles that are easy to open and close; keep door thresholds low and beveled; and avoid throw rugs.
- Carpeting and rugs should not be worn or torn, and nonskid backing should be used on loose rugs.
- Keep outside steps and railings maintained in good condition.
- Use good lighting inside and out.

- Store medications in a safe place and make sure all prescriptions are current; throw out all medications that are past the expiration date.
- Use a nonskid mat or strips on the standing area in the bathtub or shower, shower doors of safety glass or plastic, and install grab bars on the walls by the bathtub and toilet.

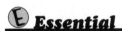
Essential

By keeping track of medications, you can avoid problems including overdosing, mixing the wrong medications, taking too many of the same type of medication, and taking the wrong medication. Compile a record that includes the name of the medication and what it's used for, directions for use, the color and shape of the pills, when it should be taken, any precautions, date of prescription, and the dispensing pharmacy.

Keeping It Clean

Clutter in homes may lead to accidents, and dust, grime, and dust mites contribute to illness and allergies. A study by the National Institute of Nursing Research showed that households that use hot water and bleach in the laundry have an almost 25 percent less incidence of infections than households that don't use bleach.

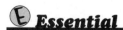

For cleaning, use a mixture of one-fourth cup of household bleach in one gallon of room-temperature water for disinfectant purposes. Apply the mixture lightly to surfaces, let it sit for ten minutes, and then rinse.

Take the following steps to help keep you safer and your home clean and hygienic:

- Take your trash out every day.
- Change your sheets at least once a week and wash all bed linens in hot water once a week to keep down the proliferation of dust mites that contribute to allergies.
- Vacuum your home frequently also to keep dust and allergies at bay.
- Seal holes and cracks in the floor and around baseboards, fireplaces, and pipes to keep dirt and insects out.
- Bathe pets once a month and keep them off couches, chairs, and beds to prevent their fur and dander from contaminating the home.

And though they seem like excellent sanitation products, keep in mind that antibacterial hand soaps wash away the good flora with the bad, so practice good handwashing techniques with mild soap and warm water instead.

Chapter 4

Common In-Home Incidents

Injuries and incidents within the home are common among all families on any given day. People get injured during everyday activities, and illnesses occur in the course of life, any of which may be mild to serious. Some are treatable at home and some require medical attention..

Cuts (Lacerations)

Cuts and abrasions of all kinds can happen every day, from scraped knees on a patio to deep cuts on fingers and hands in the kitchen and workshop. Cuts are skin wounds that involve separation of the skin and are usually caused by a sharp object like a knife or a piece of glass.

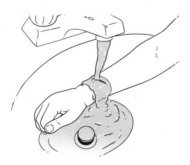

Wash cuts under running water

Take the following steps to care for simple cuts and abrasions:

1. Wash your hands with soap and water and then wash the wound under running water. For wounds that are bleeding, apply direct pressure with a sterile cloth or bandage and elevate the wound.
2. Apply antibiotic cream, but avoid using iodine or hydrogen-peroxide solutions, as they can cause further damage to injured tissues and may cause allergic reactions in people reactive to iodine and shellfish.
3. Dress the wound with a sterile gauze, preferably non-stick, bandage to protect the wound from infection and water loss until a scab forms.
4. Keep the area around the wound clean and change any dirty dressings promptly.

Change most dressings daily and replace dressings when any fluids soak through, to decrease any chance that the wound will dry and stick to the dressing. Cleaning open wounds can sometimes cause bleeding, which can be easily stopped with direct pressure using a sterile gauze pad.

Ⓔ *Alert!*

Never dress a wound with obvious contamination. If you aren't able to get it clean, then cover it lightly with a sterile bandage and seek medical attention.

First Aid for Deeper Cuts

In the case of lacerations that are deep enough to see fatty tissue:

1. Pull the edges of the wound together and use butterfly closures to secure them.
2. Apply antiseptic or antibiotic ointment over butterfly closures, cover with a bandage, and seek medical attention.

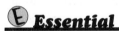

Essential

Never wash deep cuts, because it may increase the rate of bleeding. Don't remove blood-stained dressings from deep cuts, as this may restart bleeding. Instead, reinforce the old dressings by putting additional dressings on top until the bleeding stops.

See a doctor:

- For cuts that don't stop bleeding after ten minutes or applying pressure
- If there is a chance that nerves or tendons have been affected
- If there is something embedded in the cut
- If the cut is caused by an animal or human bite or was punctured by anything dirty that may cause infection
- If the cut is on the mouth, face, hand, or genitals

If stitches are needed, keep the wound closed with butterfly closures until you can get professional care. If the wound is very dirty or is likely to be so, such as with human or animal bites, you only have about six hours before the wound is too contaminated to stitch. Other wounds may go as long as eight hours after the injury before being stitched, but the longer you wait, the less likely that stitches will be possible and any scarring can be minimized. For any signs of complications such as numbness or decreased movement; tenderness, inflammation, swelling, or red streaks around the wound; or fever seek immediate medical attention.

 Fact

Call your medical-care provider immediately for wounds longer than one-half inch that are gaping open and have edges that don't stay together because as a rule these wounds need stitches.

Control the Bleeding

When a wound starts to bleed at any time, apply pressure to control the bleeding. If the cut is deep and bleeding is profuse, treat it as an emergency. Control the bleeding by placing a sterile gauze or pad over the cut and applying steady direct pressure. Lay the person down with feet elevated to help prevent shock. Never apply direct pressure to a wound with a protruding object or bone; instead, apply pressure to either side of the wound. If possible, elevate the cut above the level of the person's heart, and if bleeding is profuse and continuous, refer to Chapter 2, Managing Shock, and call 911 immediately.

First Aid for Abrasions
When treating abrasions, follow these steps:

1. Remove any debris such as dirt, fiber, and rocks from an abrasion before cleaning it.
2. Use tweezers to remove small objects, and a nonalcoholic wipe to gently clean off the wound, wiping in one direction.
3. Wash the wound with soap and water, apply an antibiotic cream, and cover with a clean dressing.

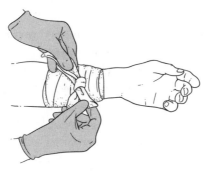

Secure a bandage with a tie

Puncture Wounds

A puncture wound is a small but deep hole caused by such things as fangs, pins, sticks, staples, nails, or any object capable of penetrating the skin deeply. Puncture wounds don't usually bleed a lot, but can cause internal injury, and it's difficult to estimate how deep the wound may be.

First Aid for Puncture Wounds

Always assume that a puncture wound is dirty. To treat minor wounds:

1. Wash your hands with soap and water and wear gloves.
2. Clean the wound under a stream of running water, using soap followed by povidone-iodine.
3. Bandage loosely and monitor the wound daily for signs of infection suh as increased swelling, redness, or discharge.

Never seal the puncture wound and do not use antibiotic ointments because sealing the wound may actually increase the chance of infection. Don't attempt to clean a major puncture wound as this may cause more serious bleeding. Never try to remove an imbedded object from a puncture wound. Depending on where the wound is located, this can cause further damage, bleeding, and even immediate death. Never probe or remove debris from a wound, attempt to push body parts back in, or breathe on a wound or dressing because doing so may cause serious infection later.

Call 911 immediately for any serious puncture wound. If the wound is bleeding heavily, apply direct pressure until help arrives.

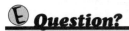

Question?

When should I change a bandage?
There are no hard and fast rules for dressing changes but typically you should change bandages daily, or whenever they get dirty or wet from activity or from blood or other secretions from the wound.

Infections Due to Cuts

There is a possibility of infection anytime the skin is broken because cuts provide an opportunity for infection-causing bacteria, viruses, and fungi to enter the body. Infections may develop only in one place on the body (localized infection) or circulate throughout the body via the bloodstream (systemic infection). Symptoms of localized infection include skin that is warm or hot, pain in the area, a pus-like discharge, redness and swelling, and fever and chills. Most minor, localized infections can be cared for at home taking the following steps:

1. Wash the area daily with soap and water.
2. Apply antibiotic ointment or cream and cover the infected area lightly with a dry gauze, nonstick bandage.
3. Watch for signs of a more serious infection such as increased redness, pain, swelling, or pus.

A localized infection may develop into a serious local infection called cellulitis, when the skin around the wound becomes raised, red, painful, and thickens in texture with symptoms including swollen lymph nodes, red streaks on the skin, fever, chills, and shaking. A local infection may also turn into a systemic infection with symptoms including fever, shaking, chills, overall weakness, and joint aches. See your medical provider if you have a localized infection that does not begin to clear in three days; for any symptoms of cellulitis or systemic infection; for any infections of the face, particularly near the eyes; for infections in young children and the elderly; or for anyone with an underlying medical condition. To prevent infection, wash hands frequently, don't pick or scratch sores or blemishes, wash all cuts or scratches with soap and water, and keep injuries clean and bandaged.

Tooth Loss, Dental Pain, and Dental Injuries

Accidental tooth loss is more common than you might think, so you may want to consider adding a tooth-preservation kit to your first-aid supplies. These kits can be found easily at most pharmacies. Cavities or infections may lead to toothaches and require a visit to the dentist, and in most cases, the sooner the better.

How to Handle Accidental Tooth Loss

A knocked-out or partially dislodged tooth can usually be reinserted in the socket within thirty minutes of an injury. Adults should hold the tooth in place with clean gauze, trying not to touch the root of the tooth. You may handle the tooth with a sterile gauze or pad and rinse it with water if it has become very dirty, but it is best not to clean a dislodged tooth. If you are not able to hold the tooth in place for any reason or you cannot reach a dentist or emergency room within thirty minutes, the tooth may be placed in a container with fresh whole milk or the person's own saliva for transport. For an empty bleeding socket, place a fold of sterile gauze or pad over the socket and bite down on it. Maintain this pressure for twenty minutes or until bleeding stops.

Alert!

> If a child loses a tooth due to accident or injury, do not try to reinsert the tooth. A child may not hold the tooth in properly or may accidentally swallow it. Instead, place the tooth in whole (not powdered or skim) milk to keep the tooth alive until a dentist can reinsert it.

Broken Teeth

Rinse the mouth with water and cover the broken tooth with a sterile gauze pad. Hold a cold pack against the face to reduce pain and swelling. Keep the broken portion and call your dentist, as the dentist may be able to reattach it. Do not eat or drink anything before receiving dental care.

First Aid for Toothache

If your tooth starts to become sensitive to cold or heat and progresses in level of pain, it's an indication that there may be gum disease or a problem related to the nerve inside the tooth. Sensitive teeth can be treated daily using a toothpaste that is designed for sensitive teeth, but if you really have a toothache you need to see a dentist.

- In the early stages of a toothache, astringent mouthwashes are antiseptic and help to shrink swollen tissue.
- Use a cold pack on the face and take aspirin, ibuprofen, or acetaminophen for pain and swelling. (Remember, never give aspirin to children younger than sixteen due to the risk of a life-threatening condition called Reye's syndrome.)
- Rub ice on your hands. According to a Canadian study, rubbing an ice cube on your hands kills tooth pain because the cold, rubbing sensation travels the same pathway to the brain as tooth pain, and overrides the signals from your mouth about half of the time. Try wrapping a cube and rubbing it where the bones of your thumb and index finger meet.
- See a dentist if the pain persists. An abscessed tooth with swelling and inflammation that is progressing from your tooth to other parts of your face is life threatening and needs immediate medical or dental care.

Diabetic Emergencies

When a person has diabetes, her body doesn't produce and properly use insulin, the hormone required by the body to convert sugar, starches, and other food into energy. Prolonged blood-sugar extremes in diabetics can cause loss of consciousness known as a diabetic coma.

What to Watch For

Symptoms of high blood sugar or low blood sugar often appear gradually and some or all of the following symptoms can signal the onset of a diabetic coma:

- Fruity-smelling breath
- Frequent urination
- Fast heart rate
- Deep and rapid breathing
- Extreme thirst
- Dry mouth
- Warm, dry, red skin
- Drowsiness
- Nausea with upper abdominal pain
- Vomiting
- Loss of consciousness
- Agitation, behavior changes, irritability

 Fact

Both hyperglycemia (very high blood sugar) and hypoglycemia (very low blood sugar) can lead to a diabetic coma, a life-threatening condition.

What to Do

In the case of hypoglycemia or hyperglycemia, take the following steps:

1. If you know the person is diabetic, or if you find a Medic Alert bracelet stating the person is diabetic, ask if she has taken her required insulin. If she has not or you are unsure, call 911 for help.
2. In the case of low blood sugar, or hypoglycemia, give her some form of sugar such as fruit juice. Don't give hard candy to someone who is very ill or in an altered state because of the risk of choking.

Many people are aware of how to treat their diabetes and how to test their blood-glucose levels. If tested blood remains below 60 mg/dL or if the person continues to have symptoms of severe hypoglycemia, hyperglycemia, or insulin reaction, call 911 and get to an emergency department.

 Essential

You should consider using an EMS notification system called "The Bottle of Life," a large medicine bottle marked on the top and sides with large red crosses. All medications and conditions are listed on a piece of paper inside the bottle and kept inside the refrigerator where first responders are trained to look for it.

Earache and Ear Injury

The most common causes of earaches are an infection of the middle ear (otitis media) and an inflammation of the outer ear canal (otitis externa), also called swimmer's ear. Causes include a minor injury to the ear canal, fluid trapped in the inner ear, or bacteria that leads to discomfort, swelling, and pain. Earaches are not contagious, and usually result from a complication to a cold and are sometimes associated with bottle feeding, pacifier use, secondhand smoke, and allergies.

Symptoms of an earache include severe stabbing pain, hearing loss, itching, fever, nausea or vomiting, swelling of the ear, ringing or buzzing sounds, and fluids draining from the ear.

First Aid for Earache

In the case of a high fever or discharge from the ear canal, get immediate medical attention, as antibiotics are necessary if the cause of the earache is an infection. Take the following steps:

- Children should always be seen by a doctor.
- Take the entire course of any prescribed antibiotics.
- Use OTC painkillers such as ibuprofen, acetaminophen, and aspirin (adults only), eardrops, and hot packs to help alleviate pain.
- To help prevent ear infections, wash hands often.
- Use a bulb syringe to suction mucus gently out of the nose of infants and toddlers and keep baby's head tilted up during feeding.

- Elevate the head of a child's bed a few inches (place item under the mattress, not on top where it could lead to suffication) to help drain the fluid that collects behind the eardrums and use a humidifier in your child's room at night.

Never place cotton-tipped swabs, matches, hairpins, or anything else in the ear. This can push wax further into the ear canal or perforate the eardrum, resulting in severe ear damage.

Treating an Ear Injury

Ear injuries are typically accompanied by pain, dizziness, hearing loss, and bleeding from inside the ear canal. Take the following steps to treat an ear injury:

1. Cover the outside of the ear loosely with a bandage or dressing to soak up blood and drainage, but do not attempt to plug the ear or try to stop any flow.
2. Place the person on the injured side with the injured ear facing down to drain the blood, and call 911 or go to an emergency department immediately.

Food Poisoning

Any activity involving food has the potential to create food poisoning or food-borne illness. Wash your hands before you start to cook or work in the kitchen and keep all food-preparation surfaces clean, using separate cutting boards for separate jobs so that you don't cross contaminate. Always wash fresh food before chopping, cutting, or eating it. When you are handling meats, follow the directions on the package labels. If you question the freshness of food in your refrigerator, then throw it out.

Food poisoning has two main categories: infective agents and toxic agents. Infective agents are mostly viruses, bacteria, and parasites. Toxic agents include such things as poisonous mushrooms, pesticides on fruits and vegetables, and improperly prepared exotic foods. Most food-poisoning cases where a specific contaminant is found are caused by viruses and bacteria. Toxic agents don't cause food poisoning as often as infectious agents do, and are usually related to an isolated episode caused by poor food preparation or something like picking wild mushrooms. When eaten, pesticides such as those found on unwashed vegetables or fruits may cause mild to severe illness with symptoms of weakness, increased salivation, blurred vision, headache, cramps, diarrhea, and shaking of the arms and legs. In recent years, some foods have been recalled by manufacturers due to contamination that has caused illnesses and even deaths.

First Aid for Food Poisoning
Use the following guidelines for treating food poisoning:

- Anyone who is experiencing short episodes of vomiting and small amounts of diarrhea that last less than twenty-four hours can be cared for at home by abstaining from solid food during the nausea and vomiting phase and drinking plenty of fluids, ideally clear liquids.

- Try to avoid alcoholic, caffeinated, or sugary drinks, and use over-the-counter rehydration products that are made specifically for children, such as Pedialyte and Rehydralyte, and sports drinks like Gatorade and Powerade diluted with water (full-strength energy drinks contain too much sugar and may worsen diarrhea) for adults.
- After nausea and vomiting have stopped and you have been able to tolerate fluids, resume eating regular food slowly beginning with plain foods such as rice, wheat cereals and breads, potatoes, bland cereals, lean meats, and baked chicken that are easy on the stomach. Unless you have lactose intolerance you can safely drink milk also.

Most of the time, you do not need an OTC medicine to stop diarrhea, but they are usually safe if used as directed and only by adults. If you have any concerns or symptoms of dehydration or nausea, vomiting, and diarrhea that last longer than twenty-four hours, bloody diarrhea and/or high fever, seek medical attention.

Allergic Reactions

An allergic reaction is an acquired, abnormal inflammatory reaction to a substance (allergen) that is usually mild to moderate in most people. Pollens, medications, certain foods, insect stings and bites, dust mites, pet dander, perfumes, and detergents may cause an allergic reaction. Allergies are common in all age groups and reactions to allergens range in severity from mild to severe to a life-threatening allergic reaction called anaphylaxis. Even though a person may previously have experienced no reactions or only very mild reactions to an allergen for many years, in some cases repeated exposures (sensitization) may eventually lead to a more severe reaction without warning. As you become more sensitized to an allergen, even a mild exposure may at some point trigger a potentially life-threatening reaction.

 Alert!

Anyone who has known serious allergies should wear a Medical Alert ID or tag and carry an epinephrine auto-injector pen with written instructions on how and when to use it. You'll need a doctor's prescription for the self-care epinephrine injector and you can call 1-800-ID-ALERT to get a medic alert bracelet.

Allergies occur when your body's defensive system, the immune system, comes into contact, by eating, touching, breathing, or injecting, with something it interprets as a foreign substance and a threat. Sometimes the immune system works to protect your body but other times it has difficulty distinguishing between the actual threats and substances that are not a threat. Those hyper-reactive systems tend to react with an inflammatory response to substances that aren't actually harmful, such as certain foods. Allergic reactions can range from mild to severe reactions requiring immediate medical attention. Sometimes symptoms are localized and immediate, but they can also be general (systemic) and delayed.

ALLERGIC REACTIONS

Skin Contact	Injection	Ingestion	Inhalation
poison plants	bee sting	medication	pollen
animal dander	medication	nuts & shellfish	dust
pollen			mold & mildew
latex			animal dander

Allergens and modes of contact

Signs and Symptoms

Most allergic reactions are mild, and although they are normally not serious or life threatening, it's a good idea to advise your doctor of the condition if it is new or unique to your medical history. The following are common symptoms of mild allergic reactions:

- Itchy skin
- Itchy, watery eyes
- Itchy, runny nose with clear nasal discharge

- Sneezing
- Rashes and hives
- Minor swelling

Mild Reactions

A localized itchy rash (contact dermatitis) can be prevented by avoiding contact with the allergen. Wash off any known allergens immediately with soap and water, keep the area clean and dry, and if needed treat with calamine lotion. For all allergy symptoms, check with your family doctor to see whether prescription or OTC allergy medication is advised, such as antihistamines, decongestants, or a combination of both. Your doctor may tell you to treat rashes with antihistamine cream or 1% hydrocortisone cream. As always, determining what is causing the allergic reaction and avoiding it is the best course of action.

Sinus Irrigation for Mild Allergies

Sinus irrigation is a method of rinsing out and irrigating the inside of your nose and the sinuses to remove any allergens. It also helps clear any areas of infection that may be forming in your nasal passages, making breathing easier, as well as moisturizing your sinuses. It's necessary to use a salt concentration similar to that of your body, or isotonic, to prevent nasal-tissue swelling and damage to the tissues. You can buy commercial products or you can make your own solution (½ teaspoon salt, ½ teaspoon baking soda, and 1 pint warm water) and store it in the refrigerator for up to two weeks.

Use the following method of sinus irrigation for relief of nasal congestion due to allergies:

1. Use a soft rubber-tip bulb syringe to irrigate the nose.
2. Stand over a sink or in the shower with head forward, mouth open, and chin out.
3. Insert the tip of the bulb syringe filled with solution in the nose, stop breathing, and squeeze the solution into nose, being careful not to swallow. If you need to swallow, stop and bend your head forward and allow solution to run out of your nose.
4. Repeat on the other side, then blow your nose very gently, closing off one side at a time and blowing with the mouth open.

If you are bothered with allergens in the air, irrigate your sinuses twice daily at first and then every day to every third day or after activities that involve being outside among allergens. You may also use a pulsating system according to the manufacturer's instructions.

 Fact

Never assume that because you or a family member has received allergy shots, you are completely protected. Families with known allergies should be especially aware of all emergency procedures, including the use of Epinephrine Auto-Injectors and CPR.

Severe Allergic Reactions

Severe allergic reactions are less common, and can be life threatening if not treated immediately. If a person is exhibiting any of the symptoms below, take them to a hospital emergency room, or call 911 for emergency transport immediately:

- Flushed face, neck, chest, arms, hands, feet, or tongue
- Swelling of the face, eyes, tongue, or lips
- Rapid breathing
- Signs of panic or anxiety
- A feeling of tightness in the chest and throat
- Abdominal cramping or pain
- Nausea and/or vomiting
- Dizziness or weakness
- Pale and damp skin
- Difficulty swallowing
- Difficulty breathing and wheezing
- Lips turning blue
- Feeling faint or loss of consciousness (LOC)

Swelling of the airway during a severe allergic reaction can result in loss of oxygen to the brain and other vital organs. If someone is experiencing these symptoms, call 911 and follow emergency-response steps as outlined in Chapter 2, as it is critical that they get immediate attention.

Anaphylactic Shock

Anaphylaxis is a sudden severe systemic (whole-body) allergic reaction that can potentially kill a person in less than fifteen minutes unless emergency measures are taken. Anaphylaxis is a constellation of symptoms including:

- Difficulty breathing
- Wheezing
- Confusion
- Abnormal breathing sounds
- Weak or rapid pulse
- Heart palpitations (missed beats)
- Blueness of the skin (including the lips and nail beds)
- Slurred speech
- Fainting
- Lightheadedness
- Dizziness
- Hives
- Itching and skin redness
- Anxiety
- Nausea and vomiting
- Diarrhea
- Nasal congestion
- Cough

Alert!

Doctors will prescribe an Epinephrine Auto-Injector for patients with severe allergies. If someone in your family has a prescription and is experiencing a severe allergic reaction in which the throat is constricting and breathing is becoming increasingly difficult, you need to use the injector immediately as instructed by their doctor.

These symptoms develop rapidly in response to an allergen, often within seconds or minutes, and without proper intervention may result in anaphylactic shock including dangerously low blood pressure, respiratory arrest (the person stops breathing), and cardiac arrest (when the heart stops beating).

Try your best to remain calm. For all severe allergic reactions, follow the steps outlined below:

1. Call 911 immediately.
2. Check for ABCs (airway, breathing, and circulation). See Chapter 2 on how to perform CPR.
3. If the person has received a bee sting, quickly and carefully scrape the stinger away with a knife, credit card, or fingernail without touching the sack that's attached (see Chapter 5). Wash the site with soap and water and apply a cold pack, keeping the sting site below the level of the person's heart if possible.
4. To prevent shock, if able to breathe easily, lay the person flat with head tilted up (do not use a pillow, as this will restrict breathing) and raise the feet eight to twelve inches. Use a blanket to keep the person warm. If the person is having difficulty breathing, place them in a sitting position and keep them calm until EMS arrive.
5. Do not give the person any food or drink if they are having difficulty breathing, swallowing, or if they are wheezing.

Chapter 5

Outdoor Events

The outdoors is a place for work, leisure, travel, and fun in all sorts of climates, weather, and conditions. Heat and cold may both have adverse consequences, and critters that live outside (or are supposed to) sometimes cause irritation or injury. Lack of proper hydration or altitude and other outdoor conditions may also cause you to feel poorly. No matter what you are doing outside, it's crucial to be aware of how to care for or give aid to people with injuries and illnesses that may result.

Animal, Human, and Insect Bites

A wide variety of insects and other critters, including humans, cause bites and stings that may be mild to moderate, uncomfortable to life threatening. It's important to know how to act, how to treat, and when to seek help for any of these potential injuries.

Scorpion Bites

Scorpions are lobster-like arthropods in the arachnid class (the same class as spiders), with a curling stinger at the end of their tail, and are usually found in desert areas of the Southwest and Mexico. Scorpion stings are not likely to be fatal and are easy to treat, but are more dangerous to children and the elderly. Symptoms include immediate pain or burning, minor swelling, sensitivity to touch, and a numb or tingling sensation.

The steps below should be followed for treating scorpion bites:

1. Wash the area with soap and water.
2. Use a cold pack on the area for ten minutes, repeating as necessary at ten-minute intervals.
3. Call the Poison Control Center for any severe symptoms.

Tick Bites

People who live near wooded and grassy areas or who spend recreation time in these locations are most susceptible to tick bites. These tiny arachnids feed on the blood of mammals such as deer, rodents, and rabbits and are able to carry disease from animal to human.

First aid for tick bites includes removing the tick immediately to avoid the bite reactions and reduce any possibility of developing one of the tick-borne infectious diseases such as Lyme disease, Colorado tick fever, and Rocky Mountain spotted fever.

To remove a tick:

1. Use a pair of flat or curved forceps or tweezers and take hold of the head of the tick as close to the skin as possible, and gently remove it without squeezing the tick.

2. Clean the area with soap and water and apply antihistamine or 1% hyrdrocortisone cream.

Get medical attention if the tick is buried too deep and you cannot remove it, you are in an area where Lyme disease is a risk, you develop fever and flu-like symptoms, or you experience muscle weakness, paralysis, or the bull's-eye rash characteristic of Lyme disease.

Alert!

Don't put petroleum jelly, alcohol, or ammonia on ticks—they will make ticks bury deeper. If you live in a high-risk area and get a tick bite, always call your doctor for advice as you may need to get additional medical care including antibiotics.

Animal Bites

Cats and dogs cause most animal bites. Cat bites can cause very deep puncture wounds and present a serious risk of infection because punctures cause bacteria to be forced deep into the skin and tissues. Dog bites also carry a risk of infection and increased incidence of damage to affected tissues. These bites usually produce marks that have broken the skin and sometimes bleeding, depending upon the severity and location of the bites. Redness and swelling typically occur within twenty-four to forty-eight hours.

For animal bites, check with a veterinarian for related health risks and have the wounds looked at by a physician. Your doctor may want to administer a tetanus shot and in some cases antibiotics. Keep the pet safe and secured in your custody until a doctor has evaluated the bite and the proper health authorities have ruled out any transmittable diseases.

For severe bites or when the injured person loses consciousness, check for airway, breathing, and circulation and begin CPR (see Chapter 2), call 911, and manage for shock until help arrives. For minor bites, take the following steps:

1. Wash your hands with soap and water and wash the bite under running water for at least five minutes.
2. Clean the bite with soap and water, saline solution, or povidone-iodine.
3. Stop bleeding with direct pressure and treat the bite as outlined for cuts and lacerations.
4. For unbroken skin, apply a cold pack.

5. Raise the wounded limb above the level of the person's heart (if possible) to reduce any swelling.
6. Check the bite site daily for signs of infection such as increased swelling, redness, or discharge.

Large and deep puncture wounds require medical attention. Always seek medical help for bites involving the neck, face, and hands due to the risk of serious infection and/or scarring.

 Alert!

Never attempt to catch a wild animal; call animal control and the police department. If it is a pet, contact the owner to find out if it has been immunized for rabies. In the case of animal bites, the animal needs to be monitored for rabies and reported to the police.

Human Bites

Human bites can be more dangerous than animal bites because of the high levels of bacteria and viruses contained in the human mouth. Human bites also have a high risk of infection. Even in minor wounds, infections can lead to complications such as severe joint infections. In the case of human bites, avoid putting the wound in your mouth because this adds bacteria to the wound. Take the following steps for human bites:

1. Use soap and water or saline to wash the wound thoroughly if the skin around the wound is not broken—never attempt to clean a wound from a human bite that is actively bleeding.
2. Apply an antibiotic ointment to the wound, cover with a nonstick bandage, and continue to watch the area carefully.
3. Seek medical attention if there is numbness or if the fingers cannot be straightened or bent.
4. If the skin is broken and bleeding, apply direct pressure with a clean, dry cloth to stop any bleeding. Elevate the area, cover the wound with a clean or sterile dressing, and seek medical help.
5. Get medical attention within twenty-four hours of being bitten in order to prevent complications from any deep wounds.

Seek medical attention for any signs of infections including warmth around the wound, swelling, pain, pus discharge, or signs of tendon or nerve damage such as inability to bend or straighten a finger and loss of sensation over the fingertip.

Spider Bites

Of the many spiders in the United States, only black-widow spider and brown-recluse spider bites are dangerous or potentially life threatening to humans. Some species of tarantula can cause serious but not life-threatening local reactions. Identifying the type of spider that has caused the bite can often aid in the treatment and may even save the person's life.

Symptoms of black-widow spider bites can appear one to twenty-four hours after the bite and include numbness at the bite site, dizziness, sweating, skin rash, intense muscle and chest pain and muscle spasms, severe abdominal cramps, nausea and vomiting, and difficulty breathing and tightness of the chest. You may also have pain at the bite site, white blisters that sometimes form painful ulcers (craters), rash, swelling and tenderness, weakness, stomach and joint pain, and fever.

Essential

If you can catch or kill the spider without endangering yourself, do so and take it with you to the emergency department, because identifying the type of spider is vital to determining the correct treatment. However, there is no antivenom for brown-recluse or tarantula bites.

First Aid for Spider Bites

The following steps should be taken for spider bites:

1. When bitten by a suspected nonpoisonous spider, wash and treat the bite site as outlined for cuts and lacerations, cover the bite with a clean dressing, and consult a doctor if any signs of infection develop.

2. For all black-widow or brown-recluse spider bites, call 911 or go immediately to an emergency department in order to receive treatment, and in the case of black-widow bites to receive antivenom.
3. Monitor the person's ABCs (see Chapter 2) and place them in a sitting position.

Snakebites

Rattlesnakes, copperhead, cottonmouth (water moccasin), coral snake, and cobras are some of the many poisonous snakes. Symptoms of a snakebite include:

- Fang marks in the skin
- Bleeding
- Blurred vision
- Warmth and burning at the sight of the bite
- Seizures
- Diarrhea
- Dizziness
- Sweating
- Fainting
- Fever
- Increased thirst
- Loss of muscle coordination
- Weakness
- Nausea and vomiting
- Numbness and tingling
- Rapid heart rate
- Severe pain at the site of the bite
- Skin discoloration and swelling

A nonpoisonous snakebite will usually produce a horseshoe-shaped ring of tooth marks on the person's skin, producing mild pain and possibly swelling. First-aid treatment of a nonpoisonous snake bite includes:

1. Washing the bite with soap and water
2. Covering the site with a sterile bandage or dressing

If you are unsure of the date of your last tetanus shot, consult with your doctor about a booster shot.

Bites that begin to swell and change color are usually indicative of a poisonous snake. Take the following steps for a poisonous snakebite:

1. Call 911 and the Poison Control Center immediately so that antivenom can be ready when the person arrives at the emergency department.
2. Calm the person, limit movement, and keep the affected area below heart level to reduce circulation of venom.
3. Remove jewelry or other constricting items and apply a loose splint to help restrict movement.
4. Monitor temperature, pulse, rate of breathing, and blood pressure if you are able. Manage signs of shock as outlined in Chapter 2.

Do not bring the dead snake in unless it can be done safely, and know that snakes can bite for up to an hour after they are dead. Don't allow the person who has been bitten to exert himself; carry him if you have to transport him. Don't apply a tourniquet or any cold compresses to the bite. Never cut into a bite or try to suction the venom by mouth. Don't allow any medications unless instructed by a doctor and don't give the person any food or drink.

Insect Stings

Insect stings only produce a mild reaction in most people. Multiple stings, stings in the mouth and throat, and stings to persons with adverse allergic reactions to the venom, however, can produce anaphylactic shock and must be treated immediately as outlined in Chapter 4.

First aid for stings includes:

1. Wash the sting site with soap and water.
2. Use a cold pack if needed to reduce swelling.
3. Keep the site of the sting below the person's heart if possible.

Additionally, using calamine lotion and Benadryl (diphenhydramine hydrochloride) can relieve itching and swelling. Also a paste of baking soda and water, or uncoated aspirin, will help reduce the stinging pain and reduce inflammation.

If the person has received a bee sting:

1. Quickly and carefully scrape the stinger away with a knife, credit card, or fingernail without touching the sack that's attached; this sack will still be pumping venom into the wound.
2. Do not use tweezers or squeeze the sack, as this may inject even more venom into the person.
3. Wash the site with soap and water and apply a cold pack, keeping the sting site below the level of the person's heart if possible.

Watch for signs of an allergic reaction that can develop up to twenty-four hours after a bee sting. If the site becomes infected, seek medical attention.

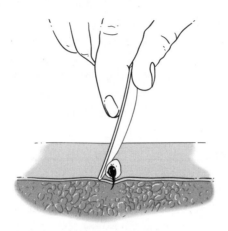

Use a credit card to scrape a stinger out

In case of allergic reaction, anaphylactic shock, or sustained multiple stings, call 911 or go to an emergency department for treatment and observation. Multiple stings can produce life-threatening reactions in otherwise healthy people.

Poison Ivy, Oak, and Sumac

More than half the people in the United States are sensitive to poison ivy, poison oak, and poison sumac and develop an itchy, blistering rash after coming in contact with these plants. Poison ivy is generally found east of the

Rocky Mountains, grows as either a vine or a shrub, and has leaves that have a smooth surface, slightly notched edges, and often clusters in groups of three. Poison oak is a small bush, sometimes a climbing vine, with smooth-edged leaves clustered in groups of three, five, or seven and more commonly found west of the Rockies. Poison-sumac leaves are generally smooth and oval shaped with seven to thirteen on each stem and grow in wet areas of the Southeast. The appearance of each of these plants can vary depending on region and seasons.

 Fact

Plant oils that are removed within ten minutes may not cause the rash. Wash thoroughly with soap and water or use rubbing alcohol to remove any oils from your skin.

Symptoms of Poison Ivy, Oak, and Sumac Rash

Exposure to any of these plants in sensitive people causes an itching rash usually appearing within twenty-four to seventy-two hours. The rash begins with small red bumps, developing into blisters of variable size later. The rash also may crust or ooze and is often in streaks (straight lines), but can take any shape or pattern, and different areas of the body can develop a rash at different times, which may make it seem like the rash is spreading.

First Aid for Poison Ivy, Oak, and Sumac Rash

Blisters may break open, but the fluid from blisters does not spread the rash; it's only spread by actual exposure to the oil that may linger on hands, clothing and shoes, or tools that act as carriers. Take special care while burning campfires in areas with poison ivy, as inhaling the smoke of a burning poison-ivy plant can be life threatening. When you are exposed to any of these plants or their oils:

1. Wash with soap and water thoroughly as soon as possible.
2. Apply cold compresses with water or milk, calamine lotion, or Aveeno oatmeal bath; and take oral antihistamines such as Benadryl (diphenhydramine hydrochloride) and 1% hydrocortisone to help alleviate symptoms.
3. For feelings of lightheadedness, lie down and raise your legs higher than your head to help blood flow to your brain.
4. If you begin to wheeze or have difficulty breathing, use an inhaled bronchodilator such as albuterol or epinephrine if it is available in order to dilate the airway, or if you have prescribed epinephrine, use it as you have been instructed.

Your doctor may also prescribe oral steroids to treat your poison ivy.

Frostbite and Hypothermia

Prolonged exposure to cold weather or brief exposure to extreme cold temperatures can result in a cold injury.

Cold injury affecting the body's shell is called frostbite, while cold injury involving the body's core is known as hypothermia. It is possible to suffer each of these separately, although they often occur simultaneously. The body's response to cold temperature is to constrict blood vessels, limiting blood flow to extremities, especially the fingers and toes, along with the release of hormones that cause shivering to increase heat production.

Frostbite

Frostbite happens when tissues freeze after exposure to temperatures below the freezing point of skin, commonly affecting the nose, cheeks, ears, fingers, and toes. Frostbite may be either superficial or deep. Symptoms of superficial frostbite include burning, numbness, tingling, itching, or cold sensations and the affected areas appear white and frozen, but if pressed on retain some resistance. Symptoms of deep frostbite include first a decrease and then a complete loss in sensation. Other symptoms include swelling, blood-filled blisters, and white or yellowish skin that appears waxy and will turn a purplish blue when rewarmed. The area will become hard with no resistance when pressed on, sometimes looking blackened and dead. Deep frostbite causes considerable pain when the blood flow is re-established and the area is rewarmed followed by a dull continuous ache and throbbing sensation in the first two to three days and lasting for weeks to months as healthy tissue separates from dead tissue.

First Aid for Frostbite

For any signs of frostbite, take the following steps:

1. Get out of the cold if you can and call for help while keeping the affected part elevated.
2. Remove jewelry and clothes that may be blocking blood flow and begin to hydrate with nonalcoholic, noncaffeinated fluids.
3. Apply a dry, sterile dressing and separate frostbitten fingers or toes with cotton, and get to a medical facility as quickly as possible.
4. Never attempt to rewarm a frostbitten area because it may freeze again and the thaw-refreeze cycle is extremely harmful.
5. Don't rub the frozen area with snow or anything else as rubbing causes further tissue damage (the amount of tissue damage is directly related to the time frozen, not to the degree of temperature).

Hypothermia

When you are exposed to cold temperatures or to cool, damp environments for prolonged periods, your body's control mechanisms may not be able to keep your body temperature normal and hypothermia can result. Hypothermia happens when your internal body temperature is less than 95°F, with gradual symptoms such as shivering, slurred speech, slow breathing, cold, pale skin, loss of coordination, fatigue, lethargy, or apathy. Children and elderly people have a higher risk of developing hypothermia.

First Aid for Hypothermia

Follow these steps for first-aid treatment of hypothermia:

1. Call 911 and monitor the person's airway, breathing, and circulation as outlined in Chapter 2 while waiting for help to arrive.
2. If you are able to, move the person out of the cold, and at the very least, attempt to protect the person from the wind and from the cold ground.
3. Remove all of the person's wet clothing and cover them with a warm, dry covering. Never apply direct heat like a hot-water bottle or heating pad; use warm packs applied to the neck, chest wall, and groin. Avoid attempting to warm the arms and legs, because the heat will force cold blood back to the heart, lungs, and brain, causing a drop in the core body temperature that can be fatal.
4. If the person is not vomiting, give them warm, nonalcoholic drinks. Handle the person gently, don't massage or rub them because a person with hypothermia is at risk of cardiac arrest.

Snow Blindness

Snow blindness is inflammation of the eyes caused when the eyes are exposed to reflected ultraviolet rays from the sun shining brightly on snow. Symptoms of snow blindness include:

- Sensation of grit in the eyes that feels worse with movement of the eyes
- Watering of the eyes
- Redness of the eyes
- Headache
- Increased pain in the eyes on exposure to light

To treat snow blindness:

1. Blindfold the person and get them to rest and avoid any further exposure.
2. If it's not possible to get the person out of the sun, protect their eyes with dark bandages or the darkest sunglasses you have.

Once out of the sun, the eyes generally heal in a few days without permanent damage. When there is any danger of snow blindness, always wear sunglasses. Don't wait to put sunglasses on until after the discomfort starts.

Dehydration

When your body is dehydrated, it doesn't have as much water and fluids as it should. Dehydration may be caused by not drinking enough fluids, losing too much fluid, or both. Depending on how much of the body's fluid is not replenished or is lost, dehydration can be mild, moderate, or severe. Severe dehydration is a life-threatening emergency. Vomiting, diarrhea, excessive urine output, excessive sweating, and fever all cause fluid loss in the body. Nausea, loss of appetite during illness, and sore throat or mouth sores may cause you to not drink enough fluids. Symptoms of dehydration include:

- Dry or sticky mouth
- Decreased or no urine output
- Urine that appears dark yellow
- Lack of tearing
- Sunken eyes
- Lethargy and coma (in severe dehydration)
- In infants, the soft spot on the top of the head (fontanelle) will be markedly sunken

Children and the elderly have a higher risk of developing dehydration.

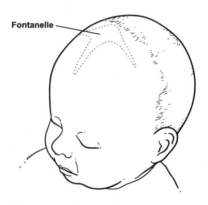

A sunken fontanelle indicates dehydration in infants

First Aid for Dehydration

You can correct mild dehydration by the following methods:

1. Frequent small amounts of fluid, rather than drinking a large amount of fluid all at once, which may cause vomiting. Electrolyte solutions are especially effective, but avoid sport drinks that contain sugar that may cause or worsen diarrhea. Also avoid plain water for rehydrating infants and children; instead, use commercial electrolyte solutions such as Pedialyte.
2. Hospitalization and intravenous fluids are sometimes necessary for moderate to severe dehydration, as well as to treat the cause of the dehydration. Call 911 for symptoms including:

   - Dizziness
   - Lightheadedness
   - Lethargy
   - Confusion
   - Lack of tears

In an infant less than two months old, diarrhea or vomiting, little or no urine output in an eight-hour period, sunken eyes, dry skin that stays up like a tent when pinched into a fold (called skin tenting), dry mouth or eyes, sunken soft spot (fontanelle), rapid heartbeat, blood in the stool or vomit, or listlessness and inactiveness.

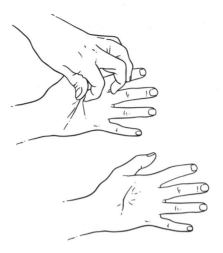

A test for dehydration is to pull on the skin and see if it stays up like a tent

Everyone should drink plenty of fluid every day and more during hot weather and while exercising. While ill, don't wait for signs of dehydration; attempt to push fluids or get medical attention.

Fact

Don't wait till you are thirsty to drink fluids. Instead stay hydrated, because it takes two hours for fluids to have any effect on your body, and by the time you feel thirsty, you are already dehydrated.

Heat Emergencies

There are three categories of heat emergencies, increasing in severity: heat cramps, heat exhaustion, and heatstroke. All three are preventable by taking precautions in hot weather. The most common causes of heat emergencies are high temperatures or humidity, dehydration, prolonged or excessive exercise, overdressing in hot temperatures, alcohol consumption, medications (particularly diuretics and psychiatric medications), cardiovascular disease, and sweat-gland dysfunction. Children, the elderly, and obese people are at increased risk of developing heat illness, but anyone can develop heat illness by ignoring warning signs.

Symptoms of Heat Illness

The early symptoms of heat illness are:

- Profuse sweating
- Fatigue
- Thirst
- Muscle cramps

Later symptoms include:

- Dizziness
- Lightheadedness
- Headache
- Weakness
- Nausea and vomiting
- Cool, moist skin
- Darkened urine

As heat illness worsens and progresses to heatstroke, the symptoms also include:

- A temperature above 104° Fahrenheit
- Irrational behavior
- Extreme confusion
- Rapid, shallow breathing
- Dry, hot, and red skin
- Weak, rapid heart rate
- Seizures
- Loss of consciousness
- Coma
- Death

First Aid for Heat Illness

For any signs of shock, seizures, or loss of consciousness, call 911 and manage airway, breathing, and circulation and shock as outlined in Chapter 2. For nonemergency cases of heat illness take the following steps:

1. Lay the person down in a cool place and elevate the feet about twelve inches.
2. To lower body temperature, apply cool water or cool, wet cloths to the skin, use a fan, and place covered cold packs on the person's neck, groin, and armpits.
3. Give the person a half cup of fluids every fifteen minutes, such as Gatorade, or a drink made by mixing a quart of cool water and a teaspoon of salt.
4. Massage cramped muscles firmly and gently.

Avoid the following:

- Don't give medications intended for fever, such as aspirin or acetaminophen, as they may be harmful in heat illness.
- Never use alcohol rubs.

- Don't give the person anything to eat or drink if they are vomiting or unconscious.
- Never give salt tablets or liquids that contain alcohol or caffeine, as they interfere with the body's mechanism of controlling internal temperature.

Never underestimate the seriousness of heat illness, particularly in children, the elderly, or injured persons. Seek medical attention for any symptoms that don't improve with intervention.

Jellyfish Stings

Jellyfish are bell-shaped, gelatinous marine creatures with tentacles that are sometimes longer than three feet. Jellyfish venom oftentimes triggers allergic reactions with symptoms including rash, intense, stinging pain, and raised welts. Symptoms may then progress to include nausea, vomiting, diarrhea, back and abdominal pain, fever, chills and sweating, and swelling of the lymph nodes. In severe reactions, a person may have difficulty breathing, slip into a coma, and even die.

First Aid for Jellyfish Stings

Anyone with severe symptoms such as intense pain, chest pain, or shortness of breath needs immediate medical attention. Call 911, manage signs of shock, and begin CPR as outlined in Chapter 2. For other reactions take the following steps:

1. Rinse the sting with seawater, not fresh water, as the latter will increase pain. Don't apply ice packs or rub the area. Irrigate eye stings with one gallon of fresh water.
2. Apply acetic acid 5% (white vinegar) or isopropyl alcohol; use one-fourth strength vinegar for mouth stings, but do not use vinegar in the case of any oral swelling or difficulty swallowing.
3. Remove any tentacles carefully with tweezers while wearing gloves.
4. Apply a paste of baking soda, mud, or shaving cream to the injury, then shave the area with a knife or razor and reapply vinegar or alcohol. The paste will prevent additional toxin discharge during the shaving.
5. Minimize movement of affected area to reduce spread of the poison. (For box jellyfish stings, wrap the extremity similar to wrapping a sprained ankle, making sure that toes and fingers are still pink, and leave bandaged until you receive medical attention.)
6. Take OTC pain relievers as directed and apply 1% hydrocortisone cream two to three times daily, or use antihistamines such as Benadryl to relieve itching.

Your doctor may prescribe topical and oral steroids, and if you continue to have redness and irritation after two to three days, it may be a sign of bacterial infection of the injury and you need to see your doctor. Be aware that allergic reactions to jellyfish stings may occur up to four weeks afterward, so watch for any signs.

Chapter 6

Anywhere Events

Everyone has minor discomforts, aches, and pains in daily life. From a tummy ache to a headache, prevention and treatment can give you relief and comfort and can help keep small problems from becoming bigger health issues. Whether you experience an accidental injury or have a chronic condition like asthma or symptom such as a fever, the key is understanding and applying the appropriate measures for prevention, management, and treatment in order to stay as healthy as you possibly can.

Burns (Thermal, Chemical, and Other)

One of the most common and most painful injuries is a burn injury. Burns are caused by extreme heat (both wet and dry), chemicals, electricity, radiation, and even extreme cold. They can affect the skin, eyes, lungs, and other internal organs. The severity of a burn is generally classified in one of three categories, based on the depth of the burn and damage.

1. First-degree burns (usually referred to as superficial burns) involve only the outermost layer of skin, called the epidermis. If treated quickly and blisters do not

form, first-degree burns usually heal very well. Sunburns are a common form of first-degree burns.

2. Second-degree burns (usually referred to as partial-thickness burns) are more serious because a deeper layer of skin is affected and because they are easily infected. Second-degree burns are the most painful because more tissue is damaged, but the nerve endings are still preserved. These burns heal well and don't require medical attention unless they are larger than two to three inches in diameter or they occur on the hands, face, buttocks, penis, or vaginal area.

3. Third-degree burns (usually referred to as full-thickness burns) are the most serious burns, involving all of the layers of the skin. In third-degree burns, the skin may appear white, black, and or leathery-looking and there may be very little pain, although the areas surrounding the burn might be extremely painful. All third-degree burns require medical treatment. Call 911 for emergency rescue and transport or take the person to the nearest emergency room.

Never apply adhesive dressings or any lotions, ointments, or creams to a first or second degree burn that you are treating at home unless the skin is broken. For any broken blisters, wash carefully with antibacterial soap and tepid water, apply antibiotic ointment, and re-bandage.

When to Call for Help

For all burns, if you are unsure of the seriousness, call 911 or go to an emergency department. All burns on children, as well as any of the following, need to be seen by a doctor:

- Third-degree burns
- Second-degree burns larger than an area the size of the palm of your hand
- First-degree burns larger than a five-palm-sized area
- Burns that extend all the way around an arm or leg
- Any "mixed" pattern of varying degrees of burns
- Burns to the genital area, face, hands, or feet

First Aid for Severe Burns

Any burned person who is experiencing dizziness or confusion, weakness, fever or chills, or shivering needs immediate medical attention. For serious burns, always call 911 first, and then perform the following steps, remembering to stay safe, assess the situation, and use universal precautions if you are able to:

1. Extinguish the cause of the burn if you are able to with water or by wrapping the injured person in a heavy towel, coat, or blanket and rolling them on the ground. Make sure none of the smoldering materials are in contact with the injured person, but don't remove any burnt clothing.
2. Check for ABCs as outlined in Chapter 2, clear the airway if necessary, and begin CPR.
3. Cool the burned area with running water as outlined for treatment of minor burns, being careful not to overcool the injured person.

4. Wait for help to arrive, or if transporting the person yourself, cover the burned area with a dry, sterile bandage or a clean nonfibrous cloth such as a sheet, not a blanket or towel, as fibers may stick to injured tissues. Don't apply ointments, creams, or lotions, and don't break any blisters.

Second-degree burns that are two inches or larger in diameter and all third-degree burns require emergency medical assistance.

Treating Minor Burns

Minor burns, or first-degree burns, and small second-degree burns can be treated properly at home with the following steps:

1. For chemical burns, remove chemical source and all clothing or jewelry having contact with the chemical.
2. Cool the burn under running water, immerse the burn in cold water, or cover it with cold packs for about fifteen to twenty minutes in order to stop the burn from damaging surrounding tissue and to reduce pain. Cover cold packs, and never apply ice directly to the skin.
3. After a first-degree burn has cooled completely, apply lotion or moisturizer to soothe and prevent dryness.
4. Cover the burn with a loosely wrapped sterile gauze bandage if necessary to keep pressure and air off the burn to reduce pain. If you can do so without causing irritation to the area, leave the burn uncovered

because minor burns heal faster and more completely when they are not covered.

5. Use OTC pain relievers such as aspirin (adults only), ibuprofen, naproxen, and acetaminophen as needed for pain.

6. For any very tender, fluid-filled blisters, you may snip a tiny hole with small scissors that have been sterilized in alcohol. For these and any broken blisters, wash carefully with antibacterial soap and tepid water, apply antibiotic ointment, and rebandage.

As minor burns heal, keep the area moisturized with skin lotion and protect the area from exposure to sunlight with clothing or a UV-proof sunscreen for a period of about a year. Areas that scar may need permanent sun protection. Most minor burns will heal in as little as a week or up to a month, and if they are treated properly, most will not scar.

 Fact

Never apply grease, oil, ointment, butter, or any other substance to any burn. Be sure to remove any clothing or jewelry from the burned area. If anything is stuck to the burn, leave it for medical professionals to remove. Immerse the burned area in cool (not ice) water to stop the heat damage to tissues near the burn.

Airway Burns

Airway burns are always serious. Call 911 as soon as possible and advise the dispatcher that you suspect an airway burn. There is potential for an airway burn if the person has burns to the head, neck, face, or torso or has been on fire or in a confined-space fire (where gases and air can become superheated). In these cases, the airway can become swollen very quickly, obstructing the flow of oxygen into the body. Signs of airway burning are usually very evident, such as:

- Soot around the nose and mouth
- Swelling and actual burning of the mouth and tongue
- Singed nose hairs
- A very hoarse voice
- Breathing difficulties

If you see signs of airway damage in a conscious person, try offering small sips of cool water to reduce swelling, and loosen clothing around the neck to improve the person's breathing. Keep the person calm until help arrives.

Treating Chemical Burns

Chemical burns are always serious, and can be life threatening. Remember that personal safety in all first-aid situations is of utmost importance. After determining safety measures:

1. Remove the person from the scene if necessary, taking steps not to become exposed to toxic fumes or liquids that are present.
2. Seal any open chemical containers and ventilate the area.
3. Call 911 and the Poison Control Center immediately.

Chemical burns usually develop much more slowly than heat-related burns, but the first-aid treatment is similar. The first symptoms are typically intense stinging pain followed by blistering, peeling, swelling, and/or discoloration of the burn site.

1. Remove any articles of the person's clothing that might have become contaminated.
2. Brush away any dry chemicals left on the body, and immediately begin pouring cold water over the burn continually for at least twenty minutes or until help arrives.
3. If you have disposable rubber gloves, use them to prevent contaminating yourself and try not to let the contaminated water you're pouring pool up on or around the person or yourself.

Chemical Eye Burns

Chemical eye burns can severely or permanently damage or destroy the eye. As with other chemical burns, wear gloves and try to prevent splashing more chemical on the person or yourself. Don't attempt (or let the injured person attempt) to touch the eye or to remove a contact lens that seems stuck to the eye.

Steps to treat a chemical eye burn include:

1. Begin washing your eye and continue for at least ten minutes. In work settings, go to the emergency eye-wash or shower station, use sterile isotonic saline solution, or if not available, use cold tap water. At home, get into the shower immediately with your clothes on in order to wash out your eye.
2. Attempt to keep your eyes as wide open as possible while using running water or eye solution to rinse them out.
3. For any alkali or hydrofluoric-acid burns, continue washing until help arrives or you are taken to an emergency department.

 Fact

Most household chemical burns in children are a result of alkali in dishwasher products. Keep all household cleaning products, paints, solvents, and other hazardous products away from children.

Look on the product label or call your regional Poison Control Center to find out the type of chemical you were exposed to. The Poison Control Center can also advise you whether to seek immediate medical care. For any pain, tearing, redness, irritation, or vision loss, or if you are unsure, go immediately to an emergency department.

Sunburn

Although sun poisoning is rarely fatal, sunburn hurts, can be disabling, and increases your risk of skin cancer. Sunburn is a burn on your skin caused by ultraviolet (UV) radiation that results in inflammation of the skin, also causing premature aging of the skin and wrinkles. Even with limited exposure to the sun, any recent exposure and prior sunburn increase your risk, although normal limited exposure to UV radiation produces beneficial vitamin D in the skin.

 Essential

Sunscreen needs to be applied thirty minutes prior to sun exposure in order to be effective. Also, regardless of what the label says, sunscreens are not waterproof and need to be reapplied in generous amounts after swimming or sweating and any sun exposure.

First Aid for Sunburn

Prevent sunburn before it starts by getting out of the sun, covering exposed skin, staying out of tanning beds, and using sunscreen with a high SPF (Sun Protection Factor). SPF indicates the time it takes to produce a skin reaction on protected and unprotected skin. For example, SPF 30, in theory, allows you to be exposed thirty times longer than without sunscreen. But this is usually not true in practice, as there is a limit to amount of sun exposure without sun damage even if applying sunscreen regularly, and people seldom apply it adequately and properly.

Take the following steps to treat sunburn:

- Use OTC pain relievers for any discomfort.
- For mild sunburn, use a cool compress with equal parts milk and water, or a cold compress with Burows Solution, which you can buy at a drugstore and use as directed.
- Moisturize with aloe-based lotions, or use juices from an aloe plant.
- Take cool (not ice-cold) baths, but avoid bath salts, oils, and perfumes to prevent sensitivity reactions.
- Don't scrub or shave the skin or use lotions with topical anesthetic medications, because you can become sensitized and allergic to the medicine.
- Stay out of the sun while you are healing, and drink plenty of fluids.

See your doctor for any severe blistering or if you are dehydrated or suffering from heat stress.

Ⓔ Alert!

Certain drugs and herbal supplements, such as sulfa drugs, antibiotics, tranquilizers, birth-control pills, arthritis painkillers, oral diabetes medications, St. John's wort, drugs for treating allergies, cancer, high blood pressure, and heart-rhythm problems, and some acne and other skin-condition treatments can increase the risk of sunburn.

Electrical Injury

When a person comes into accidental contact with an electrical energy source, an electric shock occurs that may cause injury ranging from a burn to devastating damage or death. A person who has suffered an electric shock may have very obvious severe burns or may have little to no external evidence of injury. An electrical shock has the potential to cause cardiac arrest. A brief low-voltage shock that doesn't cause any symptoms or burns of the skin doesn't require care or treatment, but for all high-voltage shocks or shocks that cause burns, go immediately to an emergency department. Children who experience electric-cord burns to the mouth need to be seen by a doctor immediately. For all critical injuries, call 911 and proceed with emergency management as outlined in Chapter 2.

Treating Electrical Burns

Electrical burns are caused when current runs through a person's body. Typically, there will be only small area burns at both the entry and exit sites, but be aware that there is likely an internal track of damage between the entry and exit burns. There may be swelling and charring at both points.

1. Call 911 immediately.
2. The person may be in shock, unconscious, or even in cardiac arrest. Check for breathing and a pulse in an unconscious person, and start CPR if necessary.

3. If the person is conscious, pour cold water over the burns until help arrives, but never pour water near a live electrical source.

Never approach a person with a suspected electrical burn until you are sure that contact with the electrical source has been broken and the current has been switched off.

Head Injuries and Head Trauma

Slipping-, tripping-, and falling-related injuries account for thousands of deaths each year and millions of disabling injuries. When someone does fall, broken bones are often the result, but sometimes falls result in a more serious injury referred to as a head trauma or head injury. In fact, head injuries from slipping, tripping, or falling are one of the most common causes of disability and death in both children and adults.

Head injuries may be mild to severe injuries that occur to the scalp and skull, such as lacerations and skull fractures, injuries to the brain and underlying tissues and blood vessels in the head. Depending on the extent of the head trauma, a head injury can also be called a brain injury, or traumatic brain injury (TBI). Concussions are head injuries that may cause immediate loss of awareness or alertness for a few minutes or a few hours after the event. Contusions are bruises to the brain that cause bleeding and swelling inside the brain in the area of impact to the head. A skull fracture is a break in the skull bone.

In head injuries that are caused by falling or a direct blow to the head, such as shaking a child, a whiplash-type injury occurs, and bruising and damage to the brain, the tissue, and blood vessels is caused when the brain jolts backward, striking the skull on one side and rebounding to strike the other side. This jarring can also cause tearing of the lining, tissues, and blood vessels, causing internal bruising, bleeding, or swelling of the brain.

Symptoms of Head Injuries

Mild head injuries do not require medical attention. The symptoms of a mild head injury may include:

- A raised, swollen area ranging from a bump or bruise to small, shallow cuts in the scalp
- Headache

Symptoms of moderate-to-severe head injury include:

- Confusion
- Loss of consciousness
- Blurry vision
- Severe headache
- Vomiting
- Slurred speech
- Inability or difficulty walking
- Dizziness
- Weakness on one side or area of the body
- Sweating, pale skin
- Seizures

- Blood or clear fluid draining from the ears or nose
- Unequal pupils
- Deep cuts or lacerations in the scalp, an open wound in the head, or a foreign object penetrating the head or skull

There also may be behavior changes including irritability and loss of short-term memory, such as being unable to accurately remember the incident or events prior to it.

First Aid for Head Injury

In the case of any signs of moderate-to-severe head injury, call 911 immediately. You can treat and care for minor head injuries safely at home, but you should always call your doctor or seek medical attention if you have any concern about how serious the head injury is. In the case of bleeding under the scalp or bruises that are outside the skull known as "goose eggs," use ice packs immediately in order to reduce swelling. Goose eggs are common and go away on their own in time. Never apply ice directly to the skin, but cover it with a cloth or towel, or use a bag of frozen vegetables wrapped in cloth or store-bought chemical ice packs and apply for twenty to thirty minutes at a time, about every two to four hours in the first twenty-four hours.

Minor injuries usually occur from heights that are less than the height of the person, and occur on a soft area like carpeting, with no loss of consciousness. For these injuries, apply ice to lessen swelling and watch the person closely, prescribe bed rest with the head elevated and give fluids and a mild pain reliever such as acetaminophen as needed. Treat any superficial cuts as outlined in Chapter 4. Any deep cuts need to be seen by a doctor and examined for any foreign matter and hidden injuries. The cuts will also be cleaned and closed with stitches, staples, or glue, and a tetanus shot will be given if the injured person has not received one in the last five to ten years.

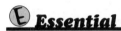

Essential

To make an ice pack, put one-third cup of 70% isopropyl alcohol and two-thirds cup of water in a plastic zip-top-style bag. This mixture will turn into a slush. You may make these packs ahead of time and freeze them to use as needed. Use crushed ice in water with small children because drinking this mixture can be poisonous.

Headache and Head Pain

Tension headaches are the most common headaches, caused by tight and rigid muscles in your shoulders, neck, scalp, and jaw, most likely due to stress, depression, or anxiety. You may suffer with tension headaches if you work too much, miss meals, or use alcohol and don't get enough sleep. Migraines, cluster headaches, and sinus headaches are also common, but whatever type of headache you suffer, it's good to know what lifestyle changes you can make, relaxation techniques you can use, and pain relievers you can take to relieve them. There are many causes of headaches, but severe headaches are less common and can signal a serious disorder. You need to inform your doctor of any sudden severe headaches, if you have a headache after a blow to the head, or if you have a headache and a stiff neck, fever, loss of consciousness, confusion, a sudden worsening in your usual pattern of headaches, or pain in the eye or ear.

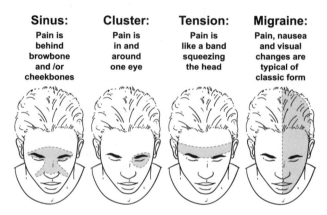

Sinus:
Pain is behind browbone and /or cheekbones

Cluster:
Pain is in and around one eye

Tension:
Pain is like a band squeezing the head

Migraine:
Pain, nausea and visual changes are typical of classic form

Types of headaches: sinus, cluster, tension, and migraine

Evaluating a Headache

In order to evaluate the cause of your headache, you need to give your doctor what is called a "headache history" by describing your headache symptoms and characteristics as completely as you are able to. Let your doctor know the following information:

- Age when the headaches started
- How frequently they occur
- If you have one or multiple types of headaches

- Frequency of headaches
- Any known triggers such as situations, foods, or medicines
- Family history of headaches
- Symptoms that occur between headaches
- If headaches affect your ability to function
- If physical activity causes or aggravates the headache
- Anything else associated with the headache

Also describe where the pain is located and what it feels like (stabbing, pounding, throbbing), the severity of the pain on a scale from 1 (mild) to 10 (severe, causing crying), how long the headaches last, if they appear suddenly without warning or with other symptoms, time of day they usually occur, and if you experience changes in vision, blind spots, or bright lights before the headache. Include any other symptoms or warning signs such as weakness, nausea, sensitivity to light or noise, appetite changes, changes in attitude or behavior, and if you have ever been treated for headaches and any medicines you are currently taking.

 Fact

Most tension headaches can be easily treated with OTC medications such as aspirin (adults only), ibuprofen, and acetaminophen. If you feel a headache coming on take a pain reliever early as they are most effective if taken before the pain gets too bad.

Migraines are more common in women, and people who have migraines may need to take prescription medication. Migraine symptoms include pain that usually affects only one side of your head, accompanied by nausea, vomiting, sensitivity to light or sound, and pain that gets worse with normal activity that can last from four to seventy-two hours.

Cluster headaches only affect 1 percent of adults, and are characterized by sudden and sharp or severe pain affecting only one side of your head, accompanied by teary eyes and nasal congestion. These headaches usually occur in a span of two to twelve weeks with one or more cluster headaches a day. Each cluster headache usually lasts forty-five to ninety minutes, leading to restlessness and pacing or rocking.

Chronic use of any medication may cause headaches known as rebound headaches, and anyone who uses medication regularly is at risk. The only treatment for rebound headaches is reducing or stopping the medication that's causing the headaches. Headaches that follow a specific activity such as exercise, sex, or bouts of coughing typically last from five minutes to forty-eight hours. This type of headache can be a sign of high blood pressure.

First Aid for Headaches

When migraines strike because of increased sensitivity to light and sound, try to rest in a quiet, dark room, and apply hot or cold compresses to your head or neck. Sometimes massage and very small amounts of caffeine will also help. Most headaches are minor and can be treated with an OTC pain reliever. For unexplained head pain or head pain that steadily worsens, call your medical-care provider. Call 911 for a headache that occurs suddenly and severely with:

- Fever
- Stiff neck
- Rash
- Changes in vision
- Dizziness
- Mental confusion

- Seizures
- Weakness
- Loss of balance
- Numbness
- Difficulty speaking

Seek medical attention for any headache that:

- Is severe following a recent sore throat or respiratory infection
- Starts or worsens after a head injury, fall, or bump
- Is a new type of pain and you are age fifty or older
- Is excruciating
- Affects just one, reddened eye
- Worsens over the course of the day
- Persists for several days

Tension headaches may be relieved by lowering body temperature by taking a cool shower. Blood vessels increase in size during headaches, and as caffeine works to constrict the blood vessels, it may be used occasionally to prevent and treat headaches. Because chronic caffeine use may cause rebound headaches, don't use it all the time. Steps to prevent and control headaches include the following:

- Keep a headache diary to help identify the cause of chronic headaches such as foods and environmental triggers.
- Avoid triggers that may include beer, wine, pickled foods, MSG, chocolate, smoked meats and cheeses, loud noises, and bright light.
- Eat a healthy diet: low fat, high in complex carbohydrates.
- Stay hydrated by drinking a cup of fluid for every twenty pounds of body weight per day.
- Eat small, frequent meals to prevent low blood sugar.
- Exercise regularly with gentle exercises such as yoga, tai chi, or swimming.
- Maintain regular sleeping hours and get seven to nine hours of sleep per night.

Ⓔ *Alert!*

Some headaches indicate serious underlying conditions. Seek emergency care if you have a headache that is sudden and severe, accompanied by a fever, stiff neck, rash, double vision, weakness, confusion, seizure, numbness, or difficulty speaking; headache following a fall or bump; or any headache that worsens even with rest and OTC pain medication.

Abdominal Pain

Abdominal pain is felt in many different ways including but not limited to burning, cramping, stabbing, throbbing, spasms, and sharp in the area below the ribs, above the pelvic bone, and around the flanks on each side. Pain in this area can arise from skin and abdominal-wall muscles but abdominal pain generally describes pain that comes from organs within the abdomen including the stomach, large and small intestines, appendix, colon, liver, gall-bladder, and pancreas. Sometimes pain that is felt in the abdomen is really coming from the lower lungs, the kidneys, and the uterus or ovaries and is called "referred" pain.

Abdominal pain is caused by inflammation, stretching or swelling of an organ, or by loss of the supply of blood to an organ. But abdominal pain can also occur without any of these causes, such as in irritable bowel syndrome (IBS). IBS is not well understood, but it may be due to abnormal contractions of the intestinal muscles (spasm) or abnormally sensitive nerves within the intestines that cause pain. Some abdominal pain is considered an emergency, such as appendicitis, or it may be a more chronic but serious condition such as diverticulitis or colitis. All abdominal pain may be serious and life threatening and needs to be evaluated by your doctor.

In children, note the following symptoms in order to describe the pain and symptoms accurately to your doctor:

- Length of time experiencing pain, particularly pain persisting for longer than twenty-four hours
- Location of pain and any pain outside the center of the abdomen
- The child's appearance, including pale skin, sweating, sleepiness, and listlessness
- Nausea and vomiting that persists for longer than twenty-four hours or vomit that appears red in color
- Diarrhea lasting longer than seventy-two hours or any blood in the stool
- Presence or absence of fever
- Groin pain (may indicate blood supply being cut off from a testicle twisting on itself)
- Urinary problems
- Any rash along with abdominal pain

After you have spoken to or been examined by your doctor, continue to monitor your symptoms or those of your child and make sure to report any changes or lack of improvement. Also be aware that depending on the age of a child, they may be reluctant to complain of symptoms.

Ⓔ Alert!

Abdominal pain is often difficult to diagnose and often takes many office visits and tests, such as blood tests, radiographic studies, and endoscopic procedures, in order to determine the problem.

First Aid for Abdominal Pain

Abdominal pain may be a sign of serious illness and can cause severe pain. You may need to describe your pain to your doctor. An easy way to think of this is that 0 is no pain and 10 is pain so severe you are crying and your face is distorted in a grimace.

0   2   4   6   8   10

Wong-Baker FACES Pain Rating Scale

Describe the pain as sharp or dull, burning or pressure like, jabbing and fleeting, steady and unrelenting or cramplike. Be sure to note any fever, chills, sweats, rectal bleeding, loss of appetite, diarrhea, weight loss, constipation, nausea, or loss of energy. Treat minor abdominal pain with:

- Rest
- A heating pad or soaking in a tub of warm water
- OTC antacids and pain relievers (but avoid aspirin or ibuprofen, as these drugs can make some types of stomach pain and conditions worse)
- Plenty of fluids and a regular diet as tolerated

For persistent pain, fever, vomiting, vaginal bleeding, loss of consciousness, chest pain, or other serious symptoms, see your medical-care provider.

Nausea and Vomiting

Everyone experiences nausea and vomiting from time to time that usually goes away quickly and can be managed at home, usually with medicine to decrease the nausea and fluid replacement for dehydration. Fluid rehydration also usually helps correct any electrolyte imbalance, which may in turn stop the vomiting.

First Aid for Nausea and Vomiting

Take the following steps to treat nausea and vomiting:

1. Hydrate with clear liquids (clear soup, broth, juice, herbal tea) beginning with small sips and increasing to four to eight ounces at a time, or one ounce or less at a time for children.
2. Avoid milk and other dairy products that may worsen nausea and vomiting.
3. After tolerating clear liquids, begin to eat soft, plain food such as oatmeal and yogurt.
4. Give children oral rehydration solutions such as Pedialyte and Rehydrate.
5. Avoid cola, tea, fruit juice, and sports drinks because they don't adequately replace fluid or electrolytes.
6. Avoid plain water, as it does not contain electrolytes and can dilute electrolytes in a dehydrated body and cause an imbalance that may lead to seizures.

If you are not able to keep fluids down, you must seek medical attention so that you can be rehydrated with an IV.

Fact

The World Health Organization has established this recipe for fluid rehydration. Mix two tablespoons of sugar or honey (only use honey for one year of age and older), one-fourth teaspoon of plain table salt, and one-fourth teaspoon of baking soda in one quart of clean or bottled water. Use this as you would any other rehydrating fluid.

Asthma Attack

Asthma affects the breathing passages of the lungs (bronchioles) due to chronic inflammation. This inflammation causes the airways of the person with asthma to become highly sensitive to a variety of "triggers," and when triggered, the passages swell and fill with mucus. This in turn causes the muscles within the breathing passages to contract or spasm (bronchospasm), which results in further narrowing of the airway passages, making it difficult for air to be exhaled from the lungs. It's this resistance to exhaling that results in the typical symptoms of an asthma attack, including wheezing, difficulty breathing, pain or tightness in the chest, anxiety, coughing, choking sensation, sweating, increased pulse, and recurrent, spasmodic coughing that is often worse during the night.

If you have asthma, you have to learn to live with the condition and be aware of any danger of attacks when exposed to something that is a trigger for you. Asthma can't be cured, but it can be controlled, particularly if it is diagnosed early and treatment is begun right away. You should always see your doctor regularly and follow your treatment recommendations. Report any changes or worsening of your symptoms and any side effects of your medications. Treatment is designed to prevent and control symptoms and asthma attacks, particularly attacks that are severe enough to require a visit to an emergency department or hospitalization.

 Fact

According to the National Institutes of Health, asthma affects more than seventeen million people in the United States that results in millions of lost days of productivity and thousands of hospitalizations every year.

Sometimes it might happen: You might have an asthma emergency. Here are some of the signs that you should look for that indicate your symptoms are getting worse:

- Sweating
- Breathing so hard that you have difficulty speaking
- Using your abdominal muscles to breathe out and skin is denting in around your ribs with breathing
- Bluish color around lips and fingernails
- Nostrils beginning to widen when breathing in
- Wheezing, breathing hard, or coughing—even after the rescue medications have been given

First Aid for Asthma

Anyone with asthma needs to be continually aware of what triggers her symptoms and to avoid those triggers, as well as how to manage symptoms. Take the following steps to help control asthma attacks:

- Identify your triggers and how you can avoid them.
- Quit smoking both cigarettes and other substances.
- Don't use any nonprescription inhalers because they are very short-acting drugs that are not likely to prevent an asthma attack and may cause undesirable side effects.
- Avoid nonprescription remedies, herbs, or dietary supplements, even those that are considered to be completely "natural" until discussing them with your doctor because some may have side effects and others may interfere with your medications.
- Don't take more asthma medication than is prescribed because overuse can also be dangerous.

In the case of an asthma attack, take two puffs of your prescribed rescue medication (inhaled beta-agonist), waiting one minute between puffs (or as recommended by your doctor), and call your doctor if you are not getting quick relief. If you are already taking oral or inhaled steroids and your treatments are not lasting four hours, you need to notify your doctor. These are only general guidelines, so always follow your doctor's instructions closely.

For any asthma attack with severe shortness of breath, call 911 immediately; do not drive yourself.

Chapter 7

Serious Incidents

Many injuries and events require basic first aid, but some also require additional assessment and special care. A small cut is relatively easy to take care of, but a serious life-threatening wound such as a gunshot wound has other critical considerations. On any given day you may be the first to happen upon a motor-vehicle accident, you may witness an accident that may have caused a spinal injury, or you may see a family member having a stroke. It's critical to know how to recognize the seriousness of all injuries, and to respond quickly, carefully, and efficiently in order to prevent further injury and to help save lives.

Bleeding

When a blood vessel or vessels are damaged, bleeding occurs. Bleeding can be external, from a cut or wound, or it can be internal, when the skin isn't broken but blood vessels inside the body are damaged. There are three different types of bleeding, depending on what kind of vessel is damaged. Arterial bleeding from damaged arteries is bright red blood that gushes in a jet with each heartbeat. Venous bleeding comes from damaged veins and causes dark red blood loss that may not be as severe but may bleed steadily. Capillary bleeding comes from tiny blood vessels found throughout the body and normally causes only slight blood loss. The seriousness of any injury depends in part on how deep a cut is, how much bleeding there is, how long it takes to control the bleeding, and the type of blood vessels that are damaged. In any bleeding injury, there is also a risk of infection, particularly if the injury results in a foreign object stuck in the wound.

 Fact

The average-sized adult has a little less than ten pints of blood and can safely lose a pint. However, any rapid loss of blood in excess of a pint will lead to a dangerous fall in blood pressure, general weakness, confusion, and sweating, also known as shock.

First Aid for Bleeding

Even though blood loss may not be severe, some people do not handle the sight of blood well, and this can cause them to behave irrationally, faint, or even go into shock.

1. Try to keep the person as calm as possible, even if it calls for mundane conversation.
2. Remember to monitor the person's ABCs and have him lie down and manage for shock if necessary (see Chapter 2).
3. Apply direct pressure to most bleeding wounds, except those that are caused by an object such as glass or those

that have protruding bone. For those types of wounds, press down firmly on either side of the object, keeping the injured body part above the level of the heart.

Controlling Severe Bleeding

Arterial bleeding may be life threatening and is often difficult to control. The first and most effective method to control bleeding is by applying direct pressure. To do this, you should:

1. Place a sterile dressing or clean cloth over the injury and secure it with tape, or tie something around the wound just tight enough to control the bleeding.
2. If bleeding doesn't stop, place another dressing over the first or apply direct pressure over the wound as outlined below.
3. Never remove a dressing once it has been applied to a severe wound.
4. Elevate an injured arm, leg, or head above the level of the heart to help control the bleeding.
5. Don't elevate or move an area of the body if you suspect a broken bone (fracture) until you have applied a splint as outlined in Chapter 9 and you are sure that movement will cause no further injury.

When the use of direct pressure and elevation are not controlling the bleeding, you can use indirect pressure by applying pressure to the appropriate pressure point. Pressure points are areas where you can control blood flow by pressing the artery against an underlying bone with your fingers, thumb, or heel of the hand. Use pressure points with caution because you may cause damage to an extremity due to inadequate blood flow from the nearby pressure. Never apply pressure to the neck (carotid) pressure points because it may reduce or stop circulation to the brain, and can also cause cardiac arrest.

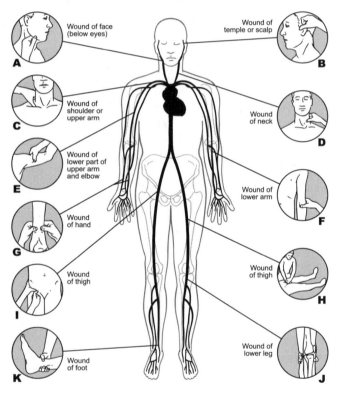

Wound of face (below eyes)

Wound of temple or scalp

Wound of shoulder or upper arm

Wound of neck

Wound of lower part of upper arm and elbow

Wound of lower arm

Wound of hand

Wound of thigh

Wound of thigh

Wound of lower leg

Wound of foot

A B C D E F G H I J K

Pressure points on the body

The two main pressure points most commonly used are in the groin and upper arm. The femoral artery starts in the lower abdomen and goes down into the thigh, and the pressure point is the front, center part of the crease in the groin that supplies the majority of blood to each leg. This artery can be found by locating the pulse on the inner part of the thigh and pressing it up against the pelvic bone.

The brachial artery is found on the upper, inside arm just below the bicep, about halfway between the shoulder and elbow. Apply pressure to the inside of the arm over the bone using your fingers or thumb. For any severe bleeding of the thigh and lower leg, place the injured person on her back, kneel on the side opposite the wounded leg, press the heel of your hand directly on the femoral-artery point, and lean forward to apply pressure. If the bleeding is still not controlled, use the flat surface of your fingertips and press directly over the artery, applying additional pressure on the fingertips using the heel of your other hand.

Tourniquets may cause tissue damage and loss of extremities and are only to be used when bleeding is uncontrollable by other methods. You can use a strap, belt, necktie, towel, or any piece of cloth folded to about three or more inches wide and six to seven layers thick. Never use anything that may cut into the skin such as wire or cord.

The steps to apply a tourniquet are:

1. Position the tourniquet between the heart and the wound while still maintaining the proper pressure point and allowing two or more inches of unharmed skin between the tourniquet and wound.

2. Put a pad or roll of gauze over the artery.
3. Wrap the tourniquet twice around the extremity and tie a half-knot (the first step in tying a shoe lace) on the upper surface.
4. Put an object like a small stick on the half-knot and complete the knot (square knot).
5. Twist the stick gently to tighten until bleeding has stopped, then secure the stick.
6. Leave the tourniquet uncovered.
7. Use marker (such as lipstick) to write a "T" on the person's forehead indicating that a tourniquet was applied, and the time the tourniquet was applied.

 Alert!

Use a tourniquet to control severe bleeding only as a last resort, and only use on the extremities. Don't loosen or remove a tourniquet after it has been applied because it may dislodge clots, resulting in continued blood loss, shock, and death.

Internal Bleeding/Blunt Trauma

You can almost always identify external bleeding, but internal bleeding is more difficult to detect and to treat. Losing blood inside the body may lead to insufficient blood flow to the tissues and organs, and dangerously low or loss of blood pressure due to insufficient volume of blood or plasma, called hypovolemic shock, which will result in death if untreated.

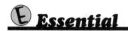
Essential

> Call your medical provider immediately for bleeding from any body opening such as the mouth, ears, nose, or rectum because it is a sign of internal bleeding that is a serious condition requiring urgent medical care.

Internal bleeding can be the result of such things as motor-vehicle accidents and domestic violence, causing internal trauma and fractures; bleeding duodenal or gastric ulcers; brain hemorrhage; and ectopic pregnancy (pregnancy occurring outside the uterus that is life threatening and requires immediate medical attention). Severe internal bleeding is usually caused by a blunt trauma, a violent force such as in motor-vehicle accidents, or from puncture wounds such as knife or gunshot wounds. Whenever signs of shock are present, you must suspect internal bleeding.

The more common signs of internal bleeding are:

- Bruises (contusions), which may indicate deeper damage
- Anxiety and restlessness
- Excessive thirst
- Nausea and vomiting
- Rapid breathing (tachypnea)
- Cold and clammy skin
- Pale ashen or bluish skin

- A rapid, weak pulse (tachycardia)
- Any bruising or discoloration at the area of injury
- Blood in the stool, or stool that appears black and tarlike
- Blood in the urine
- Swelling, distended (bloated) abdomen
- Vomiting dark red (resembling coffee grounds)
- Decreased level of consciousness
- Severe headache

First Aid for Internal Bleeding

Use the following steps to treat internal bleeding:

1. Apply a cold pack or ice pack covered with a cloth to bruises in order to reduce pain and swelling.
2. Call 911 and place the injured person with legs elevated if there is no chest injury.
3. In a case of chest injury, elevate the head and torso and keep the person warm until help arrives.
4. Manage shock as outlined in Chapter 2.
5. Don't allow the person to eat or drink or take any medication unless you are advised to do so by a doctor.

Ⓔ *Essential*

Examine the injured person for bruises, grazes, or discoloration in the chest area, markings from a seat belt, chest pain, and difficulty breathing; these may be signs of internal bleeding, so you need to be alert, as you may need to manage for shock.

Penetrating Trauma

While gunshot wounds used to be something you only saw on TV, it's a sad but true fact that these types of potentially life-threatening wounds are becoming more frequent in everyday life. Although you don't want to have the misfortune to be involved in or to witness a gunshot incident, it's vital to know how to act so that you can save a limb or even a life. Gunshot wounds and injuries caused by such things as stabbing with knives fall into the category of what is referred to as penetrating trauma.

Penetrating trauma is caused when an object pierces the skin or enters the tissue of the body, including gunshot wounds and stab wounds, as well as other types of object impalements. Penetrating injury can range from superficial punctures to penetration of major body systems, and generally the greater the speed (velocity) of penetration, the more severe the injury tends to be.

First Aid for Penetrating Trauma

Gunshot wounds and other puncture wounds like knife wounds are generally treated the same. Remember, think first of your safety and the safety of any other persons responding. In assessing the severity of a penetrating injury, it's important to understand that it may be life threatening depending on the type of object used, the location and depth of penetration, and the number of wounds. Knives and ice picks cause low-energy injuries because they are from a close distance, but one stab wound to the center of a person's chest, neck, or head with a large knife is obviously much more serious than many stab wounds with a small knife to an arm or leg.

For any penetrating injuries to the head, chest, and neck, or a wound that causes a person to fall, always suspect spinal injuries, and stabilize and protect the neck by holding the head firmly in place in line with the body. Assess for ABCs and manage as outlined in Chapter 2.

For chest wounds, note any potentially ominous symptoms, like shortness of breath and skin turning blue, along with pain in the chest and or back or the sound of airflow sucking or hissing through the puncture hole, referred to as a sucking chest wound.

At the same time, watch for any signs of what is referred to as "flail chest," where an area of the chest draws in when the person inhales, while the rest of the chest expands, and the area moves outward as the person exhales, while the rest of the chest contracts.

For a sucking chest-wound injury, follow these steps:

1. Don't remove clothing if it is stuck to the wound in a chemical environment and don't attempt to clean the wound.

2. If you can, use the person's hand to cover the wound while you get some sort of occlusive dressing together. This can be any sort of plastic wrapper, aluminum foil, or duct tape, which should be placed to extend two inches past the edge of the wound so the patch won't get sucked back into the wound, and secured with adhesive tape.

3. Only tape three sides, leaving one side untaped so that when the person exhales, air goes out of the

chest cavity and is able to escape from the open edge of the patch. When the person inhales, the patch will stick to the skin, preventing further air from entering the chest cavity (this method of patching helps to reinflate a collapsed lung).

4. Place a larger dressing loosely over the patch so it doesn't inhibit breathing, and roll the person carefully onto the injured side until help arrives.
5. Apply a thick, bulky dressing to support a flailed chest injury.

Try to check pulses at the wrist, groin, femoral, and finally the neck or carotid. If you can't feel a pulse at the carotid artery, you may need to begin CPR. Don't move the injured person unless his or her safety is in jeopardy; place unconscious persons in the recovery position as outlined in Chapter 2 until help arrives.

Don't clean up any blood on clothing, car seats, or the ground, because it's needed by first responders to estimate blood loss in order to report to the emergency department. Also, in cases of any violent crime including domestic violence, do not throw away or destroy any other evidence, including blood-stained clothing or any undergarments, obviously stained or not.

Above all, stay safe, practice universal precautions, and understand that injuries involving guns and other weapons may be in an area of potential danger to any rescuers or responders. You aren't any help to an injured person if you also get hurt. Always call 911 first if you are clear that a gun is involved. Generally, a person with a gunshot wound has a better chance of survival if they are transported to a hospital in an ambulance within ten minutes of being shot.

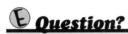

Question?

What is the "Golden Hour"?
The Golden Hour refers to the first sixty minutes after severe trauma, when it's thought that the injured person's chances of survival are greatest if he or she receives emergency care and necessary surgery.

Spinal Injury

Spinal-cord injuries are often associated with unsafe conditions such as traffic accidents, falls, rock slides, and avalanches, so it's critical for you to check the safety of the scene before helping. Call 911, and after assessing for ABCs, ask the injured person what their name is, if they know where they are and what time of day it is, and if they remember what happened, in order to determine their level of consciousness. An incorrect answer to the first three questions is an indicator of head injury and possibly a corresponding spinal-cord injury.

Any signs of drug or alcohol use or other injuries that are causing the person enough pain to ignore spinal discomfort need to be taken into consideration. Pressing lightly on a fingernail on each hand and a toenail on each foot and not seeing pink coloring return within two seconds of the release of pressure may indicate loss of circulation due to a spinal injury. Ask the person to move his fingers and toes, because difficulty moving or lack of movement indicates a spinal injury. Numbness or tingling when gently squeezing the fingers and toes also indicates possible spinal injury.

If you have any doubt, always assume a spinal-cord injury is present. You must stabilize the neck by remaining at the injured person's head, holding the neck immobile gently but firmly with one hand on each side of the head. If you have to move the person for any reason, you must logroll the person as outlined in Chapter 2. Keep the injured person's neck stabilized until help arrives.

Stroke

Strokes are a medical emergency and need immediate treatment because when blood flow to your brain stops for any reason, brain cells begin to die within a matter of minutes. The more common type of stroke is called ischemic stroke and occurs when a blood clot from any part of your body travels to and blocks a blood vessel in the brain. The second type of stroke is called hemorrhagic stroke, resulting from a blood vessel in the brain that breaks and bleeds into the brain. Transient ischemic attacks (TIA), or mini strokes, happen when the blood supply to the brain is briefly interrupted, usually for a period of about one minute but less than five minutes, and don't cause injury to the brain, due to the short duration. TIA is an important predictor of stroke.

The warning signs of a TIA or stroke are all sudden and include:

- Numbness or weakness of the face, arm, or leg, particularly on just one side of the body
- Confusion
- Trouble speaking or understanding
- Trouble seeing in one or both eyes
- Difficulty walking
- Dizziness
- Loss of balance or coordination
- Severe headache with no known cause

First Aid for Stroke

For any symptoms call 911 immediately, as prompt medical attention can prevent a fatal or disabling stroke from occurring. Then do the following:

1. Check for ABCs and start CPR if necessary.
2. Place unconscious person in the recovery position as outlined in Chapter 2.
3. Lay the person down gently, supporting his head and shoulders with a pillow or folded garment.
4. Don't give him anything to eat or drink.
5. Reassure the person that help is on the way.

Poisoning

A person may be poisoned by injecting, inhaling, coming in contact with, or swallowing a harmful substance. According to the CDC, about 2.5 million reported poisonings occur in the United States every year. A package without a warning label isn't necessarily safe. Although symptoms of poisoning often take some time to develop, if you think someone has been poisoned, don't wait for symptoms, but get that person medical help immediately.

Many household items including medicines (for example an aspirin overdose), household detergents and cleaning products, carbon monoxide, some household plants, paints, insecticides, chemicals, and even some foods can poison if a person has inadvertent exposure. Depending on the poison, symptoms will vary, but include:

- Abdominal pain
- Bluish lips
- Chest pain
- Confusion
- Cough
- Diarrhea
- Difficulty breathing
- Blurred vision
- Dizziness
- Drowsiness
- Fever
- Headache
- Heart palpitations
- Muscle twitching
- Nausea and vomiting
- Tingling and numbness
- Seizures
- Skin rash and burns
- Stupor
- Loss of consciousness
- Unusual breath odor
- Weakness

First Aid for Poisoning

Take the following steps if you suspect poisoning:

1. Check for ABCs, call 911, begin rescue breathing and CPR if necessary, and then call the Poison Control Center at 1-800-222-1222 for advice.
2. Try to identify the poison and do not make the person throw up unless you are advised to do so by the Poison Control Center (note that parents should not use syrup of ipecac at home anymore).
3. If the person vomits on their own, take measures to clear their airway, but wrap a cloth around your fingers before sweeping out the mouth and throat.
4. If the person starts having a seizure, protect them from injury by laying them down gently on a soft surface. Do not restrain the person; instead, turn the head to one side in order to keep the airway open.
5. Roll unconscious persons onto their left side in the recovery position (see Chapter 2) until help arrives.
6. Remove the person's clothes if any poison has spilled on them and flush the skin with water.

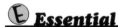 **Essential**

Call the Poison Control Center for anyone who becomes sick for no obvious reason, or is found near a furnace, car, fire, or in an area that is not well ventilated, because they need to be evaluated for poisoning.

For inhalation poisoning call 911, and only if it is safe, remove the person from the danger of the gas, fumes, or smoke. Open all the windows and doors to remove the fumes, while holding your breath or holding a wet cloth over your nose and mouth.

Drug Overdose

Drug overdoses happen when more medication is taken in higher doses or frequency than the body can metabolize. Some overdoses are accidents and some are intentional. Mixing prescription medications with street drugs and alcohol can also result in overdose. Depending on the drug taken, symptoms of overdose include:

- Slurred speech
- Abnormal breathing (slow or fast)
- Loss of coordination
- Low or high temperature
- Small (pinpoint) or enlarged pupils
- Red and flushed face
- Sweating
- Drowsiness
- Hallucinations and delusions
- Loss of consciousness
- Death

First Aid for Drug Overdose

If you think someone is having a drug overdose, perform the following first aid:

1. Check for ABCs and start CPR if necessary.
2. Manage for shock and seizures.
3. Place unconscious person in the recovery position.
4. Call 911 for any serious or life-threatening symptoms, concerns about the person's safety, or possible intention of self-harm.

Do not try to make the person throw up. Call the Poison Control Center even if the person seems to be all right. Look for pill bottles or drug paraphanelia to try to find out what the person has taken so you can give accurate information and the bottles or paraphanelia to medical providers.

Call 911 for violent or irrational behavior and take care of your own safety. Don't expect someone on drugs to be rational or try to reason with her—call for help. Try to keep your feelings and opinions separate from action, because you don't need to know why, you just need to provide first aid.

Near Drowning

Near drowning is defined as suffocation (severe oxygen deprivation) from being submerged in water that does not result in death. When death occurs, the incident is called drowning. The following are symptoms of near drowning:

- Alert, but anxious to drowsy
- Person is not breathing or is gasping for breath, coughing, or wheezing
- Vomiting
- Bluish color to the lips and ears (cyanosis)
- Pale appearance
- Cold skin

First Aid for Near Drowning

The following steps should be followed in the case of a near drowning:

1. Rescue breathing as outlined in Chapter 2 must be started at once if the person is unconscious, even while the person is still in the water, if possible.
2. If you can, ask someone else to call 911 while you begin rescue breathing.
3. Get the person safely moved to land, lay him on his back, and continue rescue breathing, beginning CPR if necessary.

Water that may gush from their mouth comes from the stomach, not the lungs, and requires that you turn the person using a log roll so that the water can drain. Vomiting can also occur.

 Fact

Many people who experience near drowning have happy outcomes. It's possible to survive a forty-minute submersion with the proper rescue and care, and many people who receive CPR and intensive care recover fully.

Providing CPR and or rescue breathing immediately will increase the chance of survival and lessen the chance and extent of any brain damage, even if you believe the person was under water for a very long time. Try to stabilize and immobilize the neck to avoid adding to any spinal injury. If the person is conscious, remove any wet clothing, then wrap him in warm blankets and get him to a hospital, regardless of how quickly you revive him or how well he may feel.

The duration of submersion under water, water temperature (cold-water accidents may have a better outcome), the person's age (children have better outcomes than adults), and how soon resuscitation begins are factors that have the most influence on a person's survival without permanent brain and lung damage. A near drowning while drinking alcohol increases a person's chances of dying or developing brain or lung damage.

Carbon-Monoxide Poisoning

Carbon monoxide is a colorless, tasteless, and odorless toxic gas that when inhaled can make you feel tired, cause headaches or dizziness, and in large amounts can lead to death. When carbon monoxide is present in the air, oxygen-carrying cells will carry the carbon monoxide rather than oxygen, and will become saturated with the gas and unable to carry needed oxygen to cells. That's why it's so important to install carbon-monoxide detectors to warn of dangerous levels.

Most carbon-monoxide poisoning cases in homes occur at night during winter months because homes tend to be sealed up tightly from the cold and may be poorly ventilated. Carbon-monoxide gas is created by the incomplete combustion of carbon-containing compounds in fireplaces, space heaters, forced-air gas furnaces, appliances, and motor vehicles that use charcoal or fuel. You are also at risk if you have any nonelectric appliances in your home, including a gas stove or water heater, or if you have an attached garage.

Common symptoms of carbon-monoxide poisoning include:

- Weakness
- Dizziness and lightheadedness
- Inability to concentrate
- Difficulty moving
- Chest pain
- Nausea
- Headache
- Shortness of breath
- Seizure
- Coma
- Irritability and lethargy in infants

 Fact

Even when awake, you may not be aware of breathing toxic fumes; only a carbon-monoxide detector can tell you for sure. They can be purchased for reasonable prices at most retail outlets and hardware stores.

First Aid for Carbon-Monoxide Poisoning

The following steps should be followed in case of carbon-monoxide poisoning:

1. If you are fortunate enough to wake up and notice symptoms of carbon monoxide poisoning, fall to the ground and crawl to an exit immediately.

2. Call 911 for the rescue of any persons left inside if you can't safely get them to fresh air yourself, and don't attempt to rescue anyone without the proper oxygen-delivering masks.
3. Get into fresh air immediately and make sure you are upwind of the house.
4. Loosen any tight clothing around your neck and waist.
5. In the case of a person losing consciousness after getting outside, maintain an open airway and begin CPR or rescue breathing as outlined in Chapter 2.

In all cases of carbon-monoxide exposure, even if you feel fine, call 911 in order to receive proper assessment and oxygen if needed.

Chapter 8

Common Conditions

Common ailments such cold and flu are sometimes accompanied by fever that may take you out of commission for a short time or cause you to miss work and social activities. Other events like nosebleeds and black eyes may be uncomfortable, but even more frightening. Learning to deal with, treat, and prevent these common conditions will also help you deal with the fear and worry some common injuries cause, and in some cases prevent larger problems from occurring.

Fever

Fevers are one way your body defends itself against many bacteria and viruses that like to live in the body's normal temperature of 98.6°F. Increasing the temperature is one way the body works to make it harder for those sorts of invaders to survive, while activating your body's immune system. A low fever is 98.8°F to 100.8°F, mild to moderate fever is 101°F to 103°F, and a high fever is 104°F and above. Causes of fever include hot weather, immunizations, bacterial and viral infections, too much time in the sun, and allergies. Symptoms that accompany a fever often include a hot, flushed face, sweating, loss of appetite, nausea and vomiting, feeling hot, body aches, constipation, or diarrhea. High fevers are sometimes associated with delirium and seizures.

Any temperatures above 105°F orally can be serious and require immediate medical attention. For children with a fever up to 101°F and a runny nose, who are also acting cranky and tired, treat as you would a cold or flu, with nonaspirin OTC medicine for fevers—such as children's or infant's acetaminophen or ibuprofen, following package directions.

How to Take a Temperature

Most thermometers today have digital readouts for oral, rectal, under the arm (axillary), and even ear canal readings. Always read the directions so you understand what the thermometer's beeps indicate and when it's time to read the thermometer. Glass mercury thermometers are no longer recommended because of the danger associated with mercury exposure or ingestion.

To taking a child's temperature rectally you should:

1. Put a dab of petroleum jelly or other lubricant on the bulb end of the thermometer. Place child on her stomach.
2. Carefully insert the thermometer one-half to one inch into the rectum.
3. Hold the thermometer and keep the child still for three minutes (don't let go of the thermometer).
4. Remove the thermometer and read as recommended by the manufacturer.

A rectal temperature is an option for persons of any age when taking an oral temperature is not possible or may be problematic.

To take an oral temperature, place the bulb end of the thermometer under the tongue, close the mouth for the recommended time (usually three minutes), remove, and read.

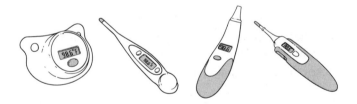

Some types of thermometers: pacifier, oral, ear, and rectal

Under the arm (axillary) temperatures are not the most accurate way to take a temperature, but if you need to use this method, you can use an oral thermometer for an armpit reading. Axillary readings are about one degree less than an oral temperature reading. Place the thermometer under the arm with arm down, and hold arms across the chest. Wait five minutes or the time recommended by your thermometer's manufacturer, remove the thermometer, and read the temperature. Seek medical attention for any of the following:

- Babies younger than three months of age with a rectal temperature of 100.4°F or higher, even with no other symptoms
- Babies older than three months of age with temperature of 102°F or higher
- Newborns with a lower-than-normal temperature, or less than 97°F rectally
- Children younger than age two with fever for longer than one day
- Children age two or older with fever for longer than three days
- Children with fever after being left in a hot car or any other hot environment—seek medical care immediately
- Adults with a temperature higher than 103°F or a fever for more than three days

Call your medical-care provider immediately for fever with any of the following:

- Severe headache
- Swelling of the throat (particularly severe swelling)

- Skin rashes
- Sudden unusual sensitivity to bright light
- Stiff neck and pain when bending the head forward or inability to bend neck forward
- Mental confusion
- Continual vomiting
- Chest pain or difficulty breathing
- Excessive listlessness or irritability
- Abdominal pain or pain during urination
- Any other symptoms of concern

 Alert!

If a fever continues to climb, or a person is not able to keep fluids down after twenty-four hours, seek medical attention.

First Aid for Fever

Take the following steps for fever:

1. Use a thermometer to monitor the temperature.
2. Remove blankets and excess clothing.
3. Keep the room cool.
4. Give sponge baths in lukewarm water.
5. Hydrate with plenty of fluids (watch for light-colored urine often, indicating a person is well hydrated).
6. Use acetaminophen to lower temperature as directed on the package.

Don't:

- Give aspirin to anyone with fever
- Use rubbing alcohol in a bath or rubbed on the skin

See your medical-care provider for any irregular breathing or shortness of breathe, stiff neck, confusion, rashes, persistent sore throat, vomiting and diarrhea, painful urination, or seizures. Fevers below 102°F in adults don't need treatment with any medications unless advised by your doctor. For fevers of 102°F or higher, take OTC medications such as acetaminophen or ibuprofen, and aspirin for ages sixteen and over only.

Febrile Seizures

Febrile seizures (convulsions) occur in children, usually due to a sudden high spike in body temperature from an infection. These seizures usually last just a few minutes, but are often startling and frightening to parents. Although they seem scary and dangerous, this type of seizure is often harmless and isn't a sign of a long-term or chronic problem. Many times the seizure occurs before an illness and fever are even recognized. Febrile seizures occur in 2–4 percent of children age six months to five years. Although fairly common and usually benign, you should seek medical attention for any febrile seizure, particularly for any necessary treatment of the underlying cause for the fever. For children prone to febrile seizures, treat fevers early to try to prevent them.

First Aid for Febrile Seizures

The signs and symptoms of a febrile seizure range from rolling of the eyes to severe shaking or tightening of the muscles. Fever is typically higher than 102°F with other signs including loss of consciousness, shaking or jerking of both arms and both legs, eyes rolling back in the head, trouble breathing, spontaneous urination, vomiting, and crying or moaning. Simple febrile seizures are the most common, usually lasting from a few seconds to fifteen minutes and stopping on their own. Take the following steps for febrile seizures:

1. Clear the area of any hard or sharp objects.
2. Lay the child down gently on a soft surface (bed or carpet), turn him on his side in order to keep the airway open, and to protect the airway in case of vomiting, place a folded jacket or pillow under his head.
3. Loosen any tight or restrictive clothing and remove any glasses.
4. Glance at your watch or a clock in order to try to time the seizure, and try to be aware of signs such as what body part is moving or twitching so that you can report this information to your doctor.
5. Call 911 for febrile seizures lasting longer than five minutes, for two or more seizures, a seizure accompanied by vomiting, or problems with breathing or extreme sleepiness after a seizure.
6. Reassure the child when he regains consciousness, and follow up with a call or visit to your doctor.

Don't:

- Try to hold the tongue or put anything in the mouth.
- Try to restrain the child; instead, turn his head to the side so that the airway does not become obstructed by his tongue or with any vomiting.
- Attempt to bring a fever down during a seizure by trying to give the child fever medications or anything to drink, and don't put the child in a bath.

When a child arouses they may cry, seem confused, or be sleepy. The severity of a seizure doesn't necessarily correlate with the degree of fever. Many children are up and running around within one to two hours of a febrile seizure. Nonetheless, have all first-time febrile seizures checked out by your doctor, no matter how short they last or how well your child seems afterward.

Seizures

Sudden, abnormal electrical activity in the brain may cause seizures. There are many different types of seizures, and some only have mild symptoms. The two main groups are focal or partial seizures that occur in just one part of the brain, while generalized seizures occur due to abnormal activity on both sides of the brain. Most seizures do not cause lasting harm and occur for thirty seconds to two minutes. Seizures lasting longer than five minutes, seizures that occur one after the other, and seizures that a person doesn't wake up between should be considered medical emergencies. Seizures have many causes, including certain diseases, medications, high fevers, and head injuries. Those with a brain disorder that causes recurring seizures have epilepsy.

 Essential

Don't put anything in a person's mouth or try to hold his tongue (it can't be swallowed during a seizure). Don't restrain the person or give liquids during or immediately after seizure. Lay the person gently on a soft surface, loosen clothing, turn his head to the side, and reassure the person when he arouses.

First Aid for Seizures

Take the following steps for someone having a seizure:

1. Lay the person down gently on a soft surface, place a folded jacket or pillow under her head, and look for any medical identification.
2. Do not restrain the person; instead, turn her head to one side in order to keep the airway open and to protect the airway in case of vomiting.
3. Loosen ties, shirt collars, and clothing, and remove any glasses.
4. Reassure the person when she regains consciousness.

For any single seizures that last less than five minutes, ask the person for any known medical history of seizure to determine if hospital evaluation is necessary. For any multiple seizures, a seizure that lasts for five minutes or more, or if the person is pregnant, injured, or diabetic, call 911.

Fainting

Fainting is a temporary loss of consciousness and muscle control causing you to fall down. Fainting is usually a result of blood pressure dropping suddenly, causing a decrease in blood flow to the brain. Some causes of fainting include heat and dehydration, emotional distress, rising from a sitting position too quickly, certain medications, a drop in blood sugar (hypoglycemia), and heart problems.

 Essential

> Most people recover from fainting quickly and completely and the cause is usually not serious, although it can be a sign of a serious problem; if you faint, you need to discuss it with your doctor.

Vasovagal syncope (fainting) is the most common cause of fainting, triggered by a stimulus that results in an exaggerated response in the part of your nervous system that regulates involuntary body functions such as heart rate and blood flow. When this response is triggered, your heart rate and blood pressure drop, reducing blood flow to your brain and causing fainting, lasting seconds to a few minutes. Some common triggers of vasovagal syncope include having a bowel movement, standing for long periods, dehydration, the sight of blood, coughing, urination, and emotional distress. Sometimes, though, there is no apparent cause.

First Aid for Fainting

If you ever feel faint, you should lie or sit down with your head between your knees. If you see someone else faint you should:

1. Place the person on her back with legs elevated above the heart if possible, to restore blood flow to the brain.
2. If the person doesn't regain consciousness after a minute, call 911.
3. Check for ABCs, begin CPR if needed, and watch for any vomiting.

Sore Throat

Sore throats are usually caused by viruses that cause colds or other upper respiratory illnesses, or bacteria, as in strep throat. Sore throats may also be caused by chemicals in such things as cigarette smoke, a scrape from something going down your throat the wrong way, allergies, postnasal drip, and sometimes cancer. Symptoms of sore throat are usually also felt throughout the body because they are present with either a viral or bacterial infection, and include fever, headache, nausea, and malaise. Signs of sore throat include pus on the surface of the tonsils, redness of the back of the throat, tender neck glands (inflamed lymph nodes), drooling and spitting due to painful swallowing, difficulty breathing, and little red blisters in the oral cavity.

First Aid for Sore Throat

The top priority for treating a sore throat is to relieve pain. This can be done in the following ways:

1. Gargle with warm salt water.
2. Take nonsteroidal anti-inflammatory drugs such as ibuprofen, aspirin (only in persons over age sixteen), and naproxen.
3. Stay hydrated by drinking enough fluids—fevers often increase fluid requirements, while painful swallowing may decrease fluid intake.

Taking pain relievers may help you increase fluid intake. Stay away from caffeine because it's very dehydrating. During cold and flu season, avoiding close contact with ill people can help keep you from getting a sore throat and other viral infections.

If you have signs of a bacterial infection, such as a severe sore throat with little coughing; a fever over 101°F along with headache, abdominal pain, or vomiting; signs of dehydration including dry mouth, sunken eyes, severe weakness, or decreased urine output; or if a family member has recently had strep throat, see a doctor immediately. If you are in such pain that you can't get to sleep with OTC medication, you should see the doctor. Go to the emergency department if swallowing causes such pain that drooling occurs, you are having extreme difficulty breathing, or you have signs of significant dehydration.

 Essential

That overall feeling of illness or malaise is your body's call for you to rest. Get as much rest and sleep as you can, drink plenty of fluids, take pain relievers as needed, and eat a good diet in order to promote more rapid recovery, particularly during a viral illness.

Croup

Croup is a type of laryngitis in children, and is associated with a seal-bark cough and difficulty inhaling air caused by swelling of the voice box (larynx) and windpipe (trachea). Croup is usually the result of a virus, but can also be caused by allergies, bacteria, or inhaled irritants. Croup is most common in children ages six months to three years, although children can get croup at any age. Croup is common during the months of October through March. Most cases today are not serious, but severe cases might require hospitalization.

Symptoms of croup are a very hoarse, deep, seal-bark-type cough appearing after several days of cold symptoms that is usually worse at night. As croup continues, a child may have labored breathing, a high-pitched squawking or crowing noise on inhalation, and a low fever. Croup is usually worst the first two or three nights, resolving in a week or so. Vaccines for measles, Haemophilus influenzae (Hib), and diphtheria protect children against the more dangerous forms of croup.

First Aid for Croup

Moist and cold air helps reduce the swelling of the airways. This can be done at home in the following way:

1. Turn the hot water on in the shower or tub of a bathroom and shut the door.
2. Once the bathroom is steamy, take your child into the bathroom and sit with him for fifteen to twenty minutes with the door closed.
3. You may also take your child, dressed warmly, out into the cold night air.

Your child should sit straight up or stand to breathe more easily. The steam treatment may help, but it doesn't cure the cough completely, so you may need to repeat this routine throughout the night each time your child wakes up coughing. You can also:

- Use a cool-mist humidifier in your child's room. (Humidifiers need to be cleaned daily with a bleach-and-water solution to prevent the growth of mold or bacteria.)
- Make sure your child is well hydrated with fluids.
- Give the appropriate dose of acetaminophen or ibuprofen for fever. Never give your child aspirin, and don't give cough medicine either; it won't help the

swelling in the throat, and it can make it more difficult to cough up mucus.

If your child is not getting any relief with steam and cold air, call your doctor for possible oral steroids to reduce swelling and help her breathe more easily. Severe cases of croup can lead to serious breathing difficulties, so call your doctor for advice if you think your child has croup. Labored breathing at rest, separate from a coughing fit, may indicate a serious, potentially life-threatening swelling in the throat. If your child is struggling for breath and drooling, and her lips or skin are turning blue, call 911 immediately.

Black Eyes

Black eyes typically occur after a blow or blunt trauma to the eye or the nose, often causing one or both eyes to swell due to the nasal injury causing fluid to collect in the thin, delicate tissues of the eyelids. Facelifts, jaw surgery, head injuries, or nose surgery may also result in black eyes. When both eyes are black and blue and swollen they are often referred to as "raccoon's eyes." (Raccoon eyes are also a sign of a type of skull fracture, so any raccoon eyes without eye trauma need to be checked out for a skull fracture.) Symptoms of black eyes are predominantly pain, bruising, and swelling. At first the swelling and discoloration may be mild, the color slightly reddened, progressing to a darker shade. As the area heals, the skin around the eye may turn a deep violet, yellow, green, or black in color, which lightens after a few days as the swelling goes down. A black eye may result in some temporary blurry vision or difficulty opening the eye because of the swelling, but lasting, serious visual problems aren't common. A black eye may be accompanied by a headache due to the blow to the head or face that caused the injury. Serious signs to watch for and report to your doctor are double vision, loss of sight, any loss of consciousness, loss of ability to move the eye, any blood or clear fluid from the nose or the ears, blood on the surface of the eye, and persistent headache.

First Aid for Black Eyes

First aid for black eyes includes the following:

1. Apply ice packs immediately after the injury in order to help decrease the swelling and pain.
2. Try to rest as much as possible.
3. Sleep with the head of your bed elevated.

Use the packs for twenty minutes of every hour you are awake during the first twenty-four hours. Be careful to wrap the ice; never apply ice directly to the skin or any area of the body. You can also use a bag of frozen vegetables wrapped in a cloth.

Stay away from all activities that may reinjure the area until after the eye has healed. Although most black eyes heal without complications, you should see an ophthalmologist to make sure that no significant injury has occurred to your eye. In addition, call your doctor for any of the following:

- Changes in vision
- Severe pain continues
- Swelling is not related to an injury
- Signs of infection such as warmth, redness, or pus-like drainage
- You are unsure about treatment or concerned about any symptoms
- You have any behavioral changes
- The swelling doesn't start to improve after a few days
- You have any swelling near the eye from a bee sting.

Go to the emergency room or your doctor immediately for any of the following:

- Changes in or loss of vision
- Inability to move your eye
- You think an object pierced your eye or is inside your eyeball
- There is any blood in your eye
- Your eye looks deformed or has fluid leaking from it
- Any cuts (lacerations) to your eye area, face, or head

You also need to go to an emergency department if you have signs of a serious head or facial injury such as:

- Broken bones or teeth
- Vomiting after the injury
- You are not able to walk after the injury
- You have blood or clear fluids coming from your nose or ears

- You take blood thinners
- You have a history of bleeding problems such as hemophilia

Broken Nose

A broken nose is a crack or fracture of the bony portion of the nose caused by trauma or a blow to the nose or face from such events as a sports injury, personal fights or domestic violence, and motor-vehicle accidents. Signs of a broken nose include tenderness when touching the nose, swelling of the nose or face, bruising of the nose or black eyes, a nose that appears deformed or crooked, nosebleed, a crunching or crackling sound or sensation when touching the nose similar to the sound that you make when you rub hair between two fingers, and pain and difficulty exhaling through the nostrils.

First Aid for a Broken Nose

Follow the steps below if you suspect a broken nose:

1. Apply an ice pack to the nose immediately for about fifteen minutes at a time and repeat multiple times throughout the day and for one to two days following the injury, to reduce pain and swelling. Make sure to take breaks between cold-pack applications, and never apply the ice directly to the skin.
2. OTC pain relievers like acetaminophen and ibuprofen can be taken as required and as directed to reduce

pain. Avoid aspirin because it may increase the chance of bleeding and swelling.
3. OTC nasal decongestants may help to aid in breathing through the nostrils.
4. Sleep with the head of your bed elevated to help with swelling of the nose.

Call the doctor if:

- The pain or swelling doesn't go away in three days
- Your nose looks crooked
- You are not able to breathe through the nose after the swelling has gone down
- You have a fever
- You begin to have frequent nosebleeds
- You feel that you have any injury that requires medical attention

Go to an emergency department immediately if:

- You have bleeding that you can't easily get under control
- You have clear fluid draining from the nose
- You have any other injuries to the face or the body
- You were knocked out
- You experience severe headaches that aren't relieved by OTC medication
- You are vomiting repeatedly
- You have a decrease or change in vision
- You have any neck pain

- You have numbness, tingling, or weakness in the arms
- You have severe pain in your nose

Nosebleed

Nosebleeds are often dramatic and frightening, but usually not serious, and are dealt with easily. The two types of nosebleeds are classified by whether the bleeding is coming from the front of the nose (anterior), accounting for 90 percent of all nosebleeds, or the back of the nose (posterior). Anterior nosebleeds are easily controlled at home or by a doctor. Posterior nosebleeds tend to occur more often in elderly people and are more complicated, often requiring hospital admission and management by an ear, nose, and throat specialist. The majority of people will experience a nosebleed at some time in their life, but they are most common in children age two to ten and adults age fifty to eighty. Nosebleeds tend to occur in the morning hours in dry, cold climates and during the winter.

Most nosebleeds are due to some identifiable factor such as allergies, blunt trauma to the nose, trauma inside the nose from such things as nose picking or irritation from a cold or cocaine use, and dry nasal passages from cold, dry air. If you have an underlying condition such as an inability of the blood to clot; are taking blood-thinning medications or aspirin; have liver disease, abnormal blood vessels or cancers in the nose, you may also experience nosebleeds. High blood pressure can also contribute to a nosebleed, but won't likely be the only cause.

Most of the time, you will only have bleeding from one nostril, but with any heavy bleeding, the blood can overflow from one nostril into the area inside the nose where the two nostrils converge and spill into the other nostril, causing bleeding from both sides. Blood can also drip into the back of the throat and be swallowed, causing you to have blood in the mouth or to even vomit blood.

First Aid for Nosebleeds

If you experience a nosebleed, follow the steps below:

1. Remain calm and sit up straight, leaning your head forward—don't tilt your head back because blood will run down your throat, causing you to gag and swallow the blood.
2. Using your thumb and forefinger, pinch your nostrils together ten full minutes, and repeat if the bleeding doesn't stop after the first ten minutes.
3. Don't swallow any blood; spit it out so that you don't vomit.

After the bleeding has stopped, try to prevent any further irritation such as sneezing or nose blowing for the next twenty-four hours.

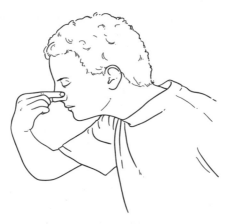

For a nosebleed, lean forward and pinch your nostrils together for ten full minutes

Don't use ice packs, because they do not help. If you have dry air in your home, like most people do in the winter, add moisture to the air with a humidifier or vaporizer or nasal gel and saline nasal spray to help keep the nose from drying out. See your doctor:

- For any repeated episodes of nosebleeds
- If you have any other bleeding, such as in the urine or stool, along with nosebleeds
- If you are bruising easily
- If you are on any blood-thinning medications
- If you have any underlying disease that may affect your blood-clotting ability, such as liver or kidney disease or hemophilia
- If you are on or have recently had chemotherapy

Alert!

Go to the emergency room if you have repeated episodes of nosebleeds during a short period of time, feel dizzy or light-headed as if you are going to pass out, you have a rapid heartbeat or any trouble breathing, or are spitting up or vomiting blood.

Motion Sickness

Motion sickness occurs when your brain gets signals that do not match the signals from your inner ears, eyes, muscles, and joints. You may experience motion sickness, also known as airsickness, carsickness, and seasickness, while traveling by car, train, airplanes, and particularly by boat or ship. Symptoms of motion sickness include dizziness, fatigue, and nausea often progressing to vomiting. Some people are naturally prone to motion sickness, and motion sickness is also associated with migraines, but others are only bothered during extreme turbulence while on a boat or plane.

First Aid for Motion Sickness

Motion sickness can be treated in the following ways:

- The best location to prevent seasickness is an interior location of a large ship, or facing forward and looking outside a ship or plane window.

- For short trips, the OTC medications meclizine, brand name Dramamine, and Bonine, are effective and can also be used for intermittent symptoms.
- On long trips, the prescription medication Transderm-Scop is a patch that can be worn behind the ear for as long as three days at a time.

Side effects of these medications are typically drowsiness, sedation, and dry mouth. Do not use motion-sickness medication if you have glaucoma or urinary obstruction.

 Fact

In studies, ginger root has been shown to be as effective as medications for motion sickness and nausea and has few to no side effects. Try taking one gram of ginger in capsule form twelve hours prior to traveling and up to four grams a day during activities that cause motion sickness.

High Blood Pressure (Hypertension)

Your blood pressure is related to the amount of blood your heart pumps and the degree of resistance to blood flow in your arteries. Even with very high, or even dangerously high, blood pressure, you don't usually have symptoms, although some people with very high blood pressure may have dull headaches, dizziness, or frequent nosebleeds.

Your risk of high blood pressure increases as you age, and although high blood pressure is more common in men, women often develop high blood pressure after menopause. Hypertension is very common among African Americans and correlates with serious complications including stroke and heart attack.

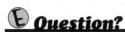

Question?

Why is high blood pressure called a silent disease?
Hypertension, or high blood pressure, is known as a silent disease because you can have it for years without any symptoms, but uncontrolled high blood pressure increases your risk of serious health problems such as heart attack and stroke.

First Aid for Hypertension

Hypertension runs in families, so it has genetic risk factors, but you can control other risk factors by increasing your level of physical activity, which helps your heart along with your waistline. The management and control of high blood pressure includes the following lifestyle modifications and medications:

- Quit smoking and keep alcohol consumption to no more than two drinks a day.
- Lose weight so that you maintain a healthy weight.
- Exercise regularly.
- Reduce sodium (salt) intake.
- Take medicines as directed.

The American Heart Association recommends a minimum of thirty minutes of exercise every other day for heart health, and the Surgeon General recommends thirty minutes of physical activity daily for overall health. Practicing stress-reduction techniques such as deep breathing and mediation, along with a healthy lifestyle, helps decrease stress and lower blood pressure.

Panic Attacks

Panic attacks can happen anywhere, anytime—while alone, in the company of others, in public, at home, and even waking you from sleep. If you have experienced a panic attack, you are aware that they are similar to an episode of extreme fear, along with the following symptoms:

- Rapid heart rate
- Sweating
- Trembling
- Shortness of breath and hyperventilation
- Chills or hot flashes
- Nausea
- Abdominal cramping
- Chest pain
- Headache
- Dizziness
- Faintness
- A feeling of tightness in your throat
- Difficulty swallowing
- A sense of impending death

Oftentimes, people experiencing a panic attack think that they are having a heart attack and seek emergency care.

Typically, a panic attack starts suddenly, peaks within ten minutes, and lasts approximately one-half hour, but some last longer, have varying patterns, and in rare cases may last up to twenty-four hours. Panic attacks may cause you to feel fatigued and worn. Anyone with frequent panic attacks has a condition called panic disorder. Panic attacks are potentially disabling, but very treatable using medications, therapy, and relaxation techniques to control or prevent the attacks. More women than men are affected by panic attacks.

First Aid for Panic Attacks

Relaxation techniques such as meditation, muscle relaxation, relaxed breathing, and guided imagery (visualization) may help keep attacks at bay and help ease signs and symptoms of stress such as headaches, anxiety, high blood pressure, trouble falling asleep, hyperventilation, and clenching or grinding of teeth. Practice focusing on relaxing your body by following these steps:

1. Sit or lie down in a comfortable position with your eyes closed.
2. Let your jaw drop and your eyelids become relaxed and heavy, but not tightly closed.
3. Starting with your toes and working up slowly to your legs, buttocks, torso, arms, hands, fingers, neck, and head, concentrate on each part individually, relaxing each area before moving on to the next.

4. In the same order, tighten the muscles in each area of your body, holding the muscle tight for a count of five and then relaxing and moving on to the next area.

Continue the process, tightening and relaxing the muscles of your face, shoulders, arms, legs, and buttocks. Don't dwell on any thoughts while you are practicing relaxation; just focus on being relaxed and calm, the fact that your hands are warm (or cool if you prefer) and heavy, that your heart is beating peacefully, and that you feel perfectly serene, while breathing deeply, slowly, and regularly.

After you feel relaxed, think of being in a place you love. After five or ten minutes of this peaceful state, you may gently rouse yourself. Practice this technique once a day until you feel you have some control over your stress.

Along with your stress-reduction techniques, it's essential to get enough sleep, eliminate caffeine, and have a regular exercise program. If your panic attacks are recurrent, you persistently worry about the attacks for a month or longer, or you feel you need to change your behavior (for example, by avoiding locations or situations in which you've previously had an attack), then you may have a panic disorder and you need to see your doctor.

Chapter 9

Emergency Events

Childbirth is a normal everyday occurrence, but when it's your responsibility to deliver a baby, it becomes an emergency. Although miscarriage may also occur frequently in the population, it is an emergency occurrence when it happens in your life. Rabies and tetanus are other life–threatening, though not everyday, events that need prompt and proper treatment. This chapter will be helpful in managing these events should they occur.

Childbirth (Emergency Delivery)

Emergency childbirth may occur in women who:

- Have had a previous rapid delivery
- Have certain connective-tissue diseases (Marfan's syndrome or Ehrlos-Danlos syndrome)
- Have a condition that makes the cervix incapable of staying closed
- Have a history of premature labor
- Have been injured or seriously ill

Emergency childbirth can also occur in otherwise healthy pregnant women who simply can't make it to the hospital on time. Should you ever be in an emergency situation with a woman who is about to give birth, it is important to understand the normal course of labor and childbirth. Labor has three stages:

- In the first stage, the uterus begins to contract in order to open and push the baby down through the birth canal.
- During the second stage, the baby is born when the mother bears down or pushes along with the contractions.
- In the third stage, the afterbirth or placenta is expelled.

 Essential

Labor generally lasts twelve to twenty-four hours for first-time moms. Subsequent births usually last three to eight hours. Because these time frames are highly variable and babies often come sooner than expected, if a woman tells you she is about to give birth, you should believe her!

First Aid for Emergency Childbirth

You should call for help as soon as possible. You may also be able to get someone on the phone to help guide you through the birth. If there is no other help around, you have no choice, and must deliver the baby yourself. Follow these steps during the first stage of childbirth:

1. Keep the mother occupied, but do not overtire her.
2. Encourage her to remain calm, relax between contractions, and breathe deeply and slowly in the midst of contractions, particularly as they become stronger. As labor progresses, she will have regular contractions that are prolonged, stronger, and closer together.
3. Prepare a place to deliver the baby that is clean and where the mother-to-be can either lie down or sit in a leaning position with her back supported.
4. When labor begins, she may experience a low backache and irregular cramping in her lower abdomen as her uterus contracts and her cervix begins to dilate. Her contractions will then become stronger and more regular, and will last longer. Assess contractions by placing your hand on her abdomen. You will feel a hardening during contractions, and can then time the interval from when the uterus begins to harden until it relaxes completely.
5. Time the intervals between the beginning of a contraction and the beginning of the next contraction— as the time decreases between contractions, her labor is progressing.
6. Sometimes standing or walking is helpful to move labor along. Let her have small amounts of food and liquids in order to give her more energy.
7. Don't try to wipe away any vaginal secretions because you may contaminate the birth canal.

If her bag of water ruptures, there will be a flow of blood-tinged mucous. The end of the first stage is commonly referred to as "transition" and is the most uncomfortable part of labor.

The mom needs your encouragement now because she may feel tired, discouraged, and irritable. She may have a lot of emotions, complain of pain and backache, may vomit and tremble, feel scared or even panicky, and she may cry and act angry. So be sure to give her lots of encouragement and reassure her that things are progressing as they should. You might help her with some relaxation techniques and some deep abdominal breathing. Encourage her to start each contraction with a deep breath to keep her body relaxed so that she will not intensify the pain and her contractions will be easier. Coach her to slow down her breathing and to breathe deeply and rhythmically. Pressing on her lower back firmly may also help relieve the backache.

Stage Two
When her cervix is almost fully opened, the baby begins to enter the birth canal as the second stage of labor begins. When this occurs, follow these steps:

1. Her contractions may come further apart and she may feel inclined to push. She should then take a deep breath with the contraction, hold her breath, and push gently. There isn't any hurry at this stage—she should rest or sleep between contractions.
2. Try to remain calm and be prepared to give any necessary first aid to both the mother and baby, such as CPR for the baby and hemorrhage control and prevention of shock for Mom.
3. Try to use sterile supplies or at least the cleanest available. You can use clean towels, clothing, or even newspaper under the mother during delivery. If she is on the ground, try to fashion some sort of covering under her, like a blanket.
4. Have her lie on her back with her knees bent and opened wide, and have her hold her knees back and apart.
5. You will see the top of the baby's head when it reaches the opening of the birth canal.
6. Ask her to pant like a dog while you apply a gentle pressure to the lower edge of the vagina as the baby's head starts to show, in order to prevent the baby from coming too fast and causing the vaginal tissues to tear.
7. Instruct her to pant, not push, until both of the baby's shoulders have been delivered.
8. As the baby emerges, support the area with a sterile gauze pad or washcloth while the head eases out.
9. Wipe the babies face with a clean or sterile cloth and quickly check around the neck for the cord.

10. If you feel the cord, hook it with your finger, pulling it around the baby's head. Some cords are wrapped one or more times around the baby's neck, so check again, and if it's too tight to slip over the baby's head, wait until the delivery is complete to untangle it.

11. After both shoulders have emerged, one at a time, the baby will slip out quickly.

12. If after several contractions a shoulder doesn't appear, slip two fingers in and feel for an armpit, hook your fingers under the armpit, and try to turn the shoulder counterclockwise as you are pulling out.

13. Cradle the head gently in your hands; don't pull or exert pressure while you guide the shoulders out.

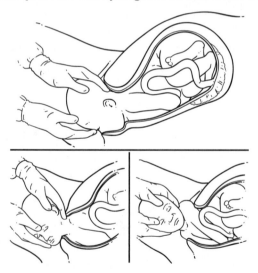

Guide the baby's head, supporting it with your hands, as it is delivered

Fact

Thousands of babies have been successfully delivered with no medical attention. If you find yourself having to assist with a birth try to remain calm and follow the outlined procedure carefully and remember that most births proceed without complications, even unaided.

Stage Three

Be aware that the baby will be very slippery, so you need to be careful not to drop it, and not to pull on the umbilical cord when picking the baby up. Instead, do the following:

1. Hold the baby at the ankles with a finger between the ankles.
2. With your other hand, hold the shoulders with the thumb, middle finger around the neck, and your forefinger on the head.
3. Hold the baby with the body a little higher than the head so that mucous and other fluids will drain from the nose and mouth.
4. Suction the mouth and nose with a bulb syringe if you have one, or use a straw to suck out the mucous or wipe it carefully with a clean cloth.
5. If the baby doesn't breathe right away, clear the mouth of mucous very gently with a bulb syringe or

your finger while gently rubbing the back. This should stimulate crying.

6. If there is still no breathing, pull the lower jaw back and give very gentle puffs at twenty puffs a minute.
7. If the baby doesn't breathe and there is no pulse, proceed with CPR as outlined in Chapter 2.
8. Clamp the cord immediately by tying a double knot with a shoelace or any other tie about four inches from the baby's umbilicus.

Fact

Do not push on the baby's head in the birth canal, hold the mother's legs together, allow a laboring mother to sit on the toilet during delivery, try to pull the baby from the vagina, or pull on the umbilical cord.

If the umbilical cord is long enough, let the mom hold her baby in her arms. If the cord is too short, you can place the baby on the mom's abdomen, gently helping to support it. Allowing the baby to breastfeed offers benefits to the baby and helps to deliver the placenta with less bleeding. As the placenta begins to appear:

1. Do not try to pull on the cord to make it come out; gently rotate it clockwise and allow it to slip out.
2. After the placenta emerges, there may also be a small amount of additional bleeding and blood clots.

3. The uterus should contract slightly and feel like a firm grapefruit just below the mother's navel. If the uterus feels soft, try to get the baby to nurse to stimulate the uterus to contract, and gently massage the uterus at the area just below the umbilicus to lessen the chances of bleeding.
4. Keep the mother flat with the foot of the bed elevated.
5. Place a cold pack on her lower tummy to help the uterus contract.
6. Using several sanitary napkins and your hand, apply pressure to the area between the anus and the opening to the vagina.
7. Watch for any symptoms of shock such as dilated pupils, faint and rapid pulse, shallow and irregular breathing, dizziness, and vomiting. For any of these signs, manage for shock as outlined in Chapter 2.
8. If there is no imminent medical help (hours or even days) after the placenta is delivered, tie another firm knot about two inches from the other knot and then cut the umbilical cord with scissors you have sterilized in boiling water or alcohol.
9. Make sure to save the placenta and any other membranes for a doctor to look at.
10. Record the estimated amount of vaginal bleeding—it should be about one to two cups.
11. Keep the mom and baby warm but not overheated, and continue to monitor the baby's color and respiration.
12. If you feel the baby has poor color or stops breathing, you may flick the soles of the baby's feet gently with a couple of fingers to encourage crying.

ⓔ *Essential*

> Don't cut the tied umbilical cord unless you are not going to have medical care for many hours. Leave it and the placenta attached to the baby to avoid potential infection to the baby.

Give the mother something to eat and drink and let her rest and hold the baby as desired. She should be free to get up and go to the bathroom, and you may also do this safely. Although almost all emergency births are normal and without complications, this is still a precarious time for the mother, as hemorrhage and shock may occur, so someone needs to stay with her at all times until she gets medical attention.

Miscarriage

A miscarriage, or spontaneous abortion, is a pregnancy that suddenly ends before the fetus can survive, and occurs in about 20 percent of all known pregnancies. Any vaginal bleeding is thought to be a potential miscarriage; however, vaginal bleeding in early pregnancy is common, and nearly one out of every four pregnant women has some bleeding in the first few months. About one half of women stop bleeding and complete their pregnancy.

A miscarriage is inevitable when there is severe bleeding along with opening of the cervix, and typically, cramping and abdominal pain. Incomplete miscarriage occurs before the twentieth week of pregnancy and bleeding is heavier, usually with abdominal pain and expulsion of some, but not all, of the products of conception; an ultrasound will show some matter still remaining in the womb. Complete miscarriage, or spontaneous abortion, is the expulsion of all products of conception, including fetus and placental tissues from the womb. Typically, abdominal pain and bleeding occur, but the discomfort and bleeding stop after the tissues and fetus have been expelled.

Causes of Miscarriage

The most common reason for miscarriages during the first three months of pregnancy (or first trimester) is an abnormal fetus, usually due to genetic problems (chromosomal abnormality), which are found in up to 70 percent of miscarried fetuses. Other reasons for miscarriage include:

- Chronic illnesses, including severe high blood pressure, lupus, and diabetes
- Thyroid problems
- Kidney disease
- Acute infections such as CMV (cytomegalovirus), mycoplasma (walking pneumonia), and German measles
- Extreme emotional shock
- Abnormal uterus
- Fibroids
- Poor muscle tone in the cervix (incompetent cervix)
- Abnormal growth of the placenta
- Multiple gestations

- Certain drugs, including alcohol, tobacco, cocaine, and possibly caffeine

First Aid for Miscarriage

Call your doctor or provider if you know or think you may be pregnant and you have any of the following symptoms:

- Vaginal bleeding
- Abdominal or back pain or cramping
- Weakness or dizziness
- Severe nausea or vomiting
- Heavy bleeding
- Severe dizziness or loss of consciousness
- A fever greater than 100.4°F
- You pass tissue
- You've had prior ectopic pregnancies

Any tissue you expel should be placed in a container and brought to the hospital. Although a miscarriage may be frightening and extremely difficult, most women are successful at completing subsequent pregnancies. You need to wait until you have recovered fully, usually a few weeks to a few months, after a miscarriage before attempting to conceive again. Many doctors recommend waiting until you've had several subsequent menstrual cycles. Take the time to work through your emotions regarding your loss, and get any professional help that you may need to help you recover.

Tetanus

Open wounds contaminated with tetanus bacteria (*Clostridium tetani*), found in soil, dust, and animal feces, can lead to a tetanus infection if you don't have up-to-date immunity. Your best defense against tetanus is prevention by vaccination, because tetanus may be fatal even with treatment. Signs and symptoms of tetanus appear from a few days to several weeks after an injury and include:

- Muscular irritability
- Spasms or stiffness of the jaw, neck, and other muscles
- Fever

Tetanus is also known as lockjaw because when the toxin spreads to the nerves of muscles, the face and jaw muscles in the area will react with strong spasms. There may also be difficulty swallowing, irritability, and difficulty breathing.

First Aid for Tetanus

For any deep or dirty wounds, see your doctor to obtain a tetanus booster shot if you haven't had a booster within the past five years, a tetanus shot in the last ten years, or aren't sure of your status. If you develop tetanus, you will most likely receive intensive treatment, and may recover completely; however, in most cases there's a risk of death or lasting effects such as brain damage despite treatment.

The tetanus vaccine is usually given to children as part of the diphtheria, tetanus, and pertussis vaccine;

teens and adults get the tetanus and diphtheria vaccine. Get the vaccine for any international travel or after any deep or dirty wounds when your vaccination status is not current. Clean and dress any wounds using an antibiotic cream or ointment.

Rabies

Rabies is a disease that affects humans who have been bitten by an animal infected with the rabies virus, and is almost always deadly in infected humans who do not receive treatment. In order to become infected, you must have contact with an infected animal and exposure to their saliva or brain or nerve tissue via open wounds in your skin or mucous membranes such as your eyes or mouth. Infected animals often appear sick, vicious, or crazy, hence the expression "mad dog." But infected animals may also seem confused, submissive, and even overly friendly or normal. The time from infection to development of symptoms is thirty to sixty days, but may range from fewer to ten days to several years. Symptoms may progress as follows:

- Pain, tingling, or itching from the bite area
- Flu-like symptoms of fever, chills, fatigue, muscle aches, and irritability
- High fever
- Confusion
- Agitation
- Seizures and coma

When extremely ill with Rabies, it's common to develop irregular contractions and spasms of the breathing muscles when around water, referred to as hydrophobia, or by feeling a little breeze, called aerophobia.

 Fact

Even the smallest bite can transmit rabies, so all bites or scratches by a rabid animal call for administration of a rabies shot. Call your medical care provider even if you are not sure, in order to be examined and evaluated for possible treatment.

First Aid for Rabies

Call your doctor, local public health department, or hospital's emergency department immediately after any exposure to a rabid animal. Treatment may involve administration of human rabies immune globulin (HRIG) and injection of the first in a series of rabies vaccines, along with treatment for serious bites wounds and a tetanus booster. You can do the following yourself:

1. Wash the wound immediately with soap, water, and an antiseptic iodine solution.
2. Get the owner's name, address, and phone number if the animal is a pet so that the animal can be monitored.

3. Contact the local animal-control authorities for any wild animals or stray dogs or cats so they can attempt to catch the animal.
4. Don't attempt to capture or subdue an animal yourself. If the animal was a bat, shut all windows in the room after everyone has been evacuated—if you can do this with no repeated exposure to the bat.

Severed Limb

No matter what the cause, a severed limb is a traumatic event for first-aid providers and for the injured person, so it is vital to remain calm and proceed with a rapid response.

The following steps should be followed for any severed limb:

1. Call 911 immediately.
2. Assess for ABCs, start CPR, and manage for shock as needed (see Chapter 2).
3. Do not apply a tourniquet; instead, control the bleeding by raising the limb and applying direct pressure.
4. Apply a sterile and secure dressing.
5. Regardless of the condition of the limb or limb fragments, wrap them in cling film or put them in a plastic bag, wrap the bag with something soft like a towel, and put it into another plastic bag containing crushed ice.
4. Label the bag with the time of the injury and the injured person's name and give it to emergency responders as soon as possible.

Never attempt to wash a severed limb or apply any antiseptic or disinfectant. Also, do not let the limb or limb fragments come into direct contact with ice. Finally, don't use anything but plastic to wrap the severed limb.

Sprains

Sprains occur when you stretch or tear the ligaments—the tough bands that connect the bones. Sudden or quick heavy lifting often causes sprains that can be mild to severe. Mild sprains can bear weight, but a severe sprain requires medical attention to determine whether it's just a sprain, a dislocation, or a fracture. Symptoms of a sprain include:

- Swelling
- Bruising or redness
- Pain during rest or when the injured muscle or the joint near the muscle is used
- Weakness of the extremity
- Complete inability to bear weight

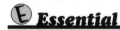
Essential

For sprains and muscle injury, use the R.I.C.E. formula: Rest, Ice, Compression, and Elevation to reduce pain and swelling and to help heal the affected muscle, tendons, ligaments, and tissues.

First Aid for Sprains

You can treat sprains at home by doing the following:

1. Apply ice packs in the first twenty-four hours and heat packs or pads when the swelling has decreased. (Note that application of heat too early will increase swelling and pain. Remember never to apply ice or heat to bare skin; only apply ice with some sort of covering, such as a towel.)
2. For pain relief and an increased ability to move around, take NSAID agents such as aspirin (for persons over sixteen only) or ibuprofen.

You may also use the R.I.C.E. formula—Rest, Ice, Compression, and Elevation—to help heal the affected muscle. This procedure entails:

1. First, ice the area for twenty minutes every hour that you are awake, for pain relief and to reduce inflammation.
2. Apply compression with an Ace or other elastic bandage wrapped firmly but not tightly, to provide support and to decrease swelling.
3. Elevate the injured area by propping up the sprain while sitting.

If your home-care methods don't give you relief after twenty-four hours, call your doctor. Go to an emergency department for any of the following:

- You hear a "popping" sound when the injury occurs
- Any significant swelling, pain or fever
- Any open cuts
- You can't walk or you lose use of an arm or leg

After the first forty-eight hours, begin to use the injured area very gently as you are able. A mild to moderate sprain should heal within two to four weeks. First aid for sprains may also be used for muscle strains.

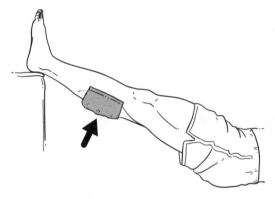

Elevate and ice a strained muscle

Broken Bones

In both children and adults, fractures are classified as open or compound when the ends of the bone have broken through the skin, raising the risk of infection. In nondisplaced fractures, the pieces on either side of the break remain lined up, and with displaced fractures the pieces of bone are not in line and may require surgery to align before casting. Hairline fractures have only a thin break in the bone, single fractures have only one break in the bone, segmental fractures have at least two and sometimes more breaks in the same bone, and in a comminuted fracture the bone is splintered or crushed.

You can identify a broken bone if you or the injured person hears, or the injured person feels, the bone break. The area will also be very tender to the touch, particularly in the area of fracture. Other signs of a broken bone include:

- Swelling around the break
- An unnatural position of the limb
- Pain on any attempts to move the limb
- Loss of a pulse below the injury
- Bone protrusion through the skin
- Abnormal movement
- A grating sensation
- Loss of function of the limb
- Bruising

Call 911 for any of the following:

- Heavy bleeding
- If even gentle pressure or movement causes pain
- Any limb or joint appears deformed
- A bone has pierced the skin
- Any extremity of an injured arm or leg is numb or bluish at the tip
- You think that a bone is broken in the neck, head, back, hip, pelvis, or upper leg

First Aid for Broken Bones

Remember to stay calm. Broken bones require medical attention, and fractures that are a result of a major trauma or injury require emergency care. Do not move the injured person, but do keep them warm.

1. Until medical help arrives, check for ABCs, treat for shock, and begin CPR if needed as outlined in Chapter 2.
2. Apply pressure to any wounds with a sterile bandage, clean cloth, or clean piece of clothing to control and stop any heavy bleeding.
3. Use covered ice packs to reduce swelling.

How to Make a Splint

If you think the bone is broken but it is not piercing the skin (closed fracture), you need to splint the limb before moving the injured person. It's important to immobilize the joint above and below where you believe the fracture site to be.

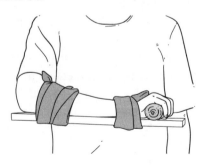

Immobilize the limb with a splint

Look around for something stiff and hard to use as a splint, such as a heavy, rigid stick. Or, you can use a rolled blanket or pack that will maintain a rigid state. If you have no other option, you can secure the injured body part to another, uninjured, body part to keep it stabilized and immobile (tape an injured finger to an adjacent, uninjured, finger).

Also keep the following in mind:

- In case of a broken bone that pierces the skin (open or compound fracture), you must apply pressure in order to control bleeding, but avoid pushing on any bone that is protruding through the skin. This is when those sanitary napkins you packed come in handy.
- Don't ever try to straighten a broken, open-fractured limb; replace bone fragments; or return the limb to a natural position.
- Don't touch or try to clean the wound; just fasten a sterile or clean pad or cloth securely in place over the wound and secure it with bandages or cloth strips (belts, scarves, neckties).
- The splint must extend beyond the injured area to keep the limb from moving. Try to cover the joint below and the joint above the injury with the splint; do not overtighten, which can cut off the circulation.
- Continue to check the area frequently for swelling, paleness, or numbness, and loosen the splint if needed.

Alert!

Do not move the injured person until a splint has been applied unless there is a greater danger of life-threatening urgency. If you do have to move a person in order to save her life, apply a splint as soon as you are able to.

Wait for professional help and continue to monitor the area, be alert for signs of shock, and keep the injured person warm. If you are not able to call for help, you must prepare to carry the person to safety.

Aftercare

Your doctor may immobilize some fractures with a splint to keep the bone from moving, kept in place with Velcro or wrapped with gauze or a bandage. Most fractured bones are placed in a cast made with either plaster of Paris or synthetic fiberglass material. For any pain in the first few days, use acetaminophen or ibuprofen, unless your pain is severe—then ask your doctor for a prescription pain medication. Sometimes there is swelling after the cast is applied, causing it to be too tight, so you need to notify your doctor immediately if your fingers or toes turn white, purple, or blue or if the skin around the edges of the cast gets red or raw, as the cast is probably too wet inside from water or sweat. Try to avoid picking at and removing any padding from the edges of fiberglass casts because the edges will then rub on the skin and cause irritation.

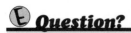

Question?

How long does it take for a broken bone to heal?
Fractures without any life-threatening complications may heal in as little as three weeks in children and four to six weeks in teens and adults. Be patient and follow the advice of your medical provider including any recommended physical therapy after the fracture has healed.

Fractures of the Pelvis

Your pelvis is the ring of bone that supports the weight of your upper body, including the two major bone commonly called hipbones. Pelvic fractures or "broken hips," however, are a common and unfortunate occurrence in the elderly. A serious pelvic fracture may also involve damage to nearby internal organs. Most pelvic fractures are the result of high-speed accidents or falls from great heights, as well as occurring during athletic activities such as hockey, skiing, football, and long-distance running. Pelvic fractures can also occur for no obvious reason or after a minor fall in elderly people, particularly due to diseases such as osteoporosis that cause the bones to weaken.

The main symptom of a pelvic fracture is groin, hip, or lower-back pain that may worsen when moving the legs. Other symptoms include:

- Abdominal pain
- Bleeding from the vagina
- Numbness or tingling in the groin, legs, urethra (urine tube), or rectum
- Difficulty urinating

Stress fractures that occur during jogging also often cause pain in the buttocks or thighs.

First Aid for Pelvic Fractures

If you suspect a serious pelvic fracture, due to witnessing a high-velocity accident or high fall for instance, call 911. Follow the steps outlined below until help arrives:

1. Don't attempt to move the injured person, particularly if the person is in severe pain or has any signs of possible nerve injury such as numbness.
2. Cover the person with a blanket or something similar in order to maintain body heat.

After being transported to the hospital and treated, it may take a few weeks to several months to heal, depending on the severity of the fracture. Treatment for minor fracture is often bed rest and OTC or prescription painkillers. The person may also need physical therapy and have to use crutches, and may sometimes require surgery.

Dislocations

An injury that forces the ends of your bones from their normal position is a dislocation. Dislocations are usually a result of some sort of trauma, such as a fall or a blow, but they can also be a result of an underlying disease such as rheumatoid arthritis. Contact sports like football and hockey, and those that may result in falls, like downhill skiing and volleyball, have a high occurrence of dislocation injuries. Dislocations happen in both major joints like the shoulder, hip, knee, elbow, or ankle and in smaller joints like fingers, thumbs, or toes. This sort of injury causes temporary deformity and inability to move the joint, usually along with sudden and severe pain. Dislocations need immediate medical attention.

First Aid for Dislocations

Get medical attention as soon as possible with any suspected dislocation so that you can have the bones repositioned properly. Until you can get medical attention, do the following:

1. Splint and immobilize the affected joint and never try force it back into place, which can potentially damage the joint, surrounding muscles, ligaments, nerves, or blood vessels.
2. Apply an ice pack to reduce any swelling caused by internal bleeding and the buildup of fluids around the injury.

Smoke Inhalation

Structural fires cause a large number of smoke-inhalation-related deaths each year. Often, people don't develop symptoms of smoke inhalation for twenty-four to forty-eight hours after the fire, and may not be diagnosed or treated correctly and in a timely manner. Inhaled smoke may cause damage to the body such as burns to the tissues in the mouth, nose, and upper respiratory system from the hot air. Some substances in smoke can be toxic to cells or can cause damage by contact with tissues. Smoke may also harm the body by interfering with the oxygen supply by preventing oxygen from reaching cells, causing cell and tissue death.

Signs and symptoms of smoke inhalation include the following:

- Singed nose hairs
- Burns on the throat and inside the nose
- Swelling of the throat
- Coughing
- Hoarseness
- Black or gray saliva
- Fluid in the lungs resulting in noisy breathing
- Shortness of breath
- Bluish-gray or cherry-red skin color
- Respiratory arrest and loss of consciousness

First Aid for Smoke Inhalation

Check for ABCs, begin CPR if needed, and manage for shock as outlined in Chapter 2. In addition:

1. Make sure the person is getting enough oxygen by taking steps to open the airway.
2. A person with smoke inhalation can get worse quickly, so exercise caution when deciding whether to transport the person to a hospital yourself—when in doubt, call 911.
3. Call 911 for anyone who has a hoarse voice, difficulty breathing, long coughing spells, or mental confusion.

Those with moderate symptoms and prompt treatment tend to recover completely, but some people may develop chronic respiratory or pulmonary (lung) disorders, particularly people with existing respiratory problems such as asthma.

Chapter 10

One for the Road

Everyone's safety on the road depends on obeying the law, maintaining vehicles, being prepared, and never driving while impaired. However, someday you may be driving and either witness or come upon the recent aftermath of an accident. Or, even worse, you may be involved in an accident yourself. You may be uninjured, but others may have mild to serious injuries, or there may even be fatalities. Steam could be rising from vehicles, there could be a smell of radiator fluid and gasoline, or there could even be smoke and fire. Some accident scenes are gruesome and shocking, but by being prepared you can quickly assess the scene and intervene to help the injured, prevent further injuries, and possibly avert deaths.

First Steps of a First Responder
The first step to take at an accident of any kind is to stop, take a few deep breaths, and perform a complete 360-degree sweep of the accident scene and your surroundings. Remember, your safety is key, so be sure to assess any safety issues before you proceed. Keep yourself safe by following these steps:

1. Park your vehicle in a safe spot that's out of the way of any other moving vehicles, being careful not to block traffic.
2. Check for any visible fuel or potentially combustible liquid on the ground, and make sure to park a safe distance away if you find any.
3. Look for any downed power lines to avoid, put on your emergency brake and your hazard lights, and call 911.
4. Check for traffic and exit your vehicle.

Do not run across any busy traffic lanes; you will not be able to help if you also become injured.

Approaching the Accident and Taking Charge
Your next steps should be:

1. Bring the first-aid kit from your vehicle and quickly but carefully approach the scene while scanning and assessing
2. Shout, "I'm here to help, is anyone hurt?"
3. Ask the first person you see how many passengers he thinks are involved.
4. If everyone visible appears unconscious or unresponsive, do a fast visual scan of the surrounding area for additional people that may have been ejected as you move around vehicles.
5. If there are other adults with you or nearby, take charge and ask for help as you need it in the most assertive way you can, without raising panic in others.

It's vital that professional rescuers and medical teams be on the way, so if you have not been able to call 911, ask someone else to call or go for help. Use common sense if you need to leave the scene to summon help yourself. Note if there are unmoving persons in the vehicles. If a small fire or heavy smoke is coming from the front of a car, threatening any passengers inside, then remove the persons from danger (without endangering yourself) before going for help. Above all else, summoning help and enlisting help in all your actions is a top priority.

It's important to note and be aware that people have a legal right to refuse medical care and that includes the right to refuse your help. Again, act appropriately for the situation, but remember that "no" means "no" in a courtroom.

Safety Measures at the Scene

In order to remain safe you must stay at least fifteen yards away from any downed power lines and always assume that they are live. Power lines that are touching any objects may also charge that object, and you may receive a fatal shock just being too close. Stop immediately if you feel any tingling sensations, put your feet together, and hop or shuffle away from the area, being very careful not to touch anything.

If a vehicle is on its side and is unstable, try to stabilize it, but only if it's necessary for your safety and/or the safety of those injured. Instruct everyone in the area not to smoke. If you are able to reach inside safely, turn off ignition switches and apply emergency brakes. If hoods are accessible and there is no indication of fire, carefully open the hood and remove the battery cable if you can.

It's very important that you never move an injured person unless you feel they will die if they are not moved. Always assume that an injured person has a neck injury and attempt to stabilize their head by placing one hand on each side of it so the head stays in line with the spine and doesn't move until help arrives.

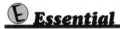 **Essential**

When you are a first responder and EMS arrives, get out of their way but remain available to answer questions and render additional assistance if they ask for it. Because you were first on the scene, you may have life-saving information to give EMS!

Sharing the Calm

One of the most important things you can do for an injured person is to reassure them and give them the impression that you are calm, even if you don't really feel that way. A violent accident and its aftermath can be emotionally traumatic, but in the moment, you must try to compartmentalize and put away any sense of fear or horror in order to help injured people as best as you can. People have been known to survive injuries that everyone on the scene believed were fatal. It is possible that a critically injured person may either fight for life and survive, or give up hope and expire, based at least in part on what they believe you think of their situation, so act confidently.

Your Personal Aftermath

Responding to a major accident with serious, sometimes fatal, injuries may be emotionally traumatic, even though at the time it may have been exciting and adrenaline pumping. Many people, even professionals, experience a wide range of delayed emotional responses when the event is over. Post-traumatic stress disorder (PTSD) is a condition that may develop after a terrifying ordeal involving physical harm, the threat of physical harm, or after witnessing a harmful event. You may experience the following symptoms of PTSD:

- Startling easily
- Feeling emotionally numb
- Losing interest in things you used to enjoy
- Having trouble feeling and expressing affection (emotional numbing)
- Irritability
- Aggressiveness or acting out in violent ways
- Reliving the trauma (flashbacks) in thoughts during the day and in nightmares during sleep

Symptoms typically begin within three months of the event, but it's possible to have symptoms years later. The course of PTSD also varies, and some people recover fully after six months, some have symptoms for a longer period, and in some, PTSD will be a chronic condition.

There are many programs designed to help you cope with PTSD that will lead to fewer and less-intense reactions, and allow you to manage trauma-related emotions with greater confidence. Some interventions include talking to your doctor about your trauma and your symptoms, talking to another person for support, practicing relaxation methods, learning how to increase positive distracting activities, talking to a counselor, and prescribed medications.

Negative coping actions such as isolation, use of drugs or alcohol, working too hard or too much, unhealthy eating, violent behavior, anger and rage, and different types of self-destructive behavior will only perpetuate the problem, increase symptoms, and further decrease your quality of life.

Keep a Useful Kit in the Car

In order to be prepared for any event, from splinters to major accidents, when on the road it's important to keep a comprehensive first-aid kit in your vehicle. The best way to decide what you might need to include involves taking a few minutes to try and imagine various conditions and scenarios you might experience where you regularly travel. Are there mountains and cliffs? Are there bodies of water next to the roads? Are the roads lighted at night? Do you travel or live in a remote location with unreliable cell-phone coverage? What is the weather like throughout the year? In addition to the items listed in Chapter 1 for your in-home first-aid kit, and depending on where you typically drive and the condition of the vehicle you drive, the following items may be useful additions to your vehicle first-aid kit:

- Large, wide-lens flashlight
- Penlight
- Several triangle reflectors
- Reflective vest(s)
- Small, multipurpose fire extinguisher
- Road flares
- Prepaid and fully charged cell phone
- Durable, multi-purpose gloves
- Several yards of coiled rope
- Duct tape
- Bungee cords
- Space blankets
- All-purpose scissors
- Note pad, pencil, and fluorescent marker
- Adjustable wrench
- A few small sand bags
- Extra batteries
- Automated External Defibrillator (AED)
- Hand sanitizer
- Flares
- CB radio
- Extra water bottles
- Walkie-talkies
- A disposable camera

Carry Insurance Cards and Medical History

When you are on the road, make sure to always carry current medical-insurance cards and updated medical histories for everyone that rides with you. If you are in an accident or someone becomes critically ill in the car, having the necessary information will help you get the right care from first responders to emergency-room medical providers.

 Alert!

The Health Insurance Portability and Accountability Act (HIPAA) guarantees your privacy in regard to medical records. If you carry medical records in your vehicle, include a note that emergency medical personnel have your permission to access and transport the information.

Good Samaritan Laws in Your State

Because of today's litigious society, there may be a certain reluctance to help out in emergency situations. Due to the fear of liability that may stop someone from getting involved, each state has laws or regulations known as Good Samaritan laws to protect you from any liability related to rescues or rescue attempts. The intent of Good Samaritan laws is to protect those who come to the aid of others for no other reason than good will, without any expectation of reward. If your daily job is some type of rescue worker, then you are accountable for any mistakes and aren't covered under Good Samaritan laws, because it is expected that you know what you are doing and that should do a good job.

Depending on the state you live in, if you help someone at an accident and afterward are rewarded monetarily or otherwise, your Good Samaritan protection may be excluded. So the way to ensure protection from any liability when helping others during rescue situations is to always act on behalf of the injured party with no expectation of reward. If you want primarily to be a hero, not to help out a fellow human being, then you risk making typical mistakes not covered by Good Samaritan laws.

Some general expectations of Good Samaritan laws are that you perform first aid to the best of your ability, and that once you have stepped forward and accepted responsibility for helping, you do not leave until other qualified help is on the scene and has relieved you. Of course, if you feel that your own life is in danger, you have the freedom to leave, and if you are performing CPR and you simply must stop from utter exhaustion, you may also stop without fear of reprisal. Good Samaritan laws may not protect you from every possible event, but they do take into account that it's human nature to make mistakes, and they do protect against reasonable mistakes. However, in that "reasonable" may be difficult to define, some people who think they should be covered under the Good Samaritan law may find themselves being sued. Ultimately, those lawsuits don't usually get to court, and if they do, they tend to lose.

How Safe Is Your Car?

Motor-vehicle accidents injure millions of people and are the cause of death for over a million people worldwide each year. Drunk driving, speeding, and improper use (or lack of use) of safety or seat belts are the leading causes of motor-vehicle accident injuries that lead to death. Motor-vehicle accidents have multiple causes including impaired driving, multitasking while driving, aggressive driving, equipment failure, and roadway maintenance and design problems.

Safety Belts and Seats

Everyone in a moving vehicle should use age appropriate restraints, including pregnant women, in order to ensure safety and be in compliance with the law. Children that are age twelve and under and those weighing less than eighty-five pounds should ride in the back seat, as airbags, which are primarily located in the front, are only designed to protect adults and have the potential to injure children. Some cars are equipped with child-safety locks that prevent a child from accidentally opening the doors from the inside.

Your local department of transportation authority has detailed instructions and laws for child safety in motor vehicles. All babies who are under twenty pounds and twelve months old must be placed securely in a rear-facing car seat in the back seat. This system has been designed to prevent severe head injuries or death, which can occur if the car seats are in the wrong position, or located in the front when an air bag deploys. Everyone should refer to specific local and state regulations for the transport of infants.

Toddlers between twenty and forty pounds and who are at least one year old can sit in a forward-facing car seat with harness straps in the back seat. Studies are also showing that it is safer to use rear-facing seats up to the age of four or five. Children who are less than 4'9" tall should sit in a booster seat. In cars with back seats that are lower than the child's ears, use a high-back booster seat for better head and neck protection. In cars with seat backs that are higher than the child's ears, use a backless booster seat. For all car seats, follow all manufacturer recommendations and instructions and never deviate from them.

Motor-Vehicle Safety

For motor-vehicle safety, always follow your vehicle operation and maintenance recommendations. Most auto manufacturers recommend oil changes every three months or three thousand miles, whichever comes first. Find a good mechanic to keep your car in tip-top shape with regular tune ups if you are not able to work on it yourself. Check your tire pressure at least once a month to prevent unexpected flats, and make sure to rotate your tires and check their alignment at your regular tune ups or every other oil change.

Pay attention to warning signs, such as things that don't feel, sound, or smell right or if you find leaks or stains where you park. Don't forget that an ounce of prevention is worth a pound of cure, particularly when it may lead to an auto-related injury. Get your vehicle ready for the changing seasons, because defending your auto against the elements will lessen your chances of weather-related accidents and roadside problems and will even fend off costly repairs. Learn the basics of caring for your vehicle so that you can check your fluids regularly. If you are able to, keep your car in a garage, or do your best to keep it in a dry, temperate place in order to keep interior and exterior wear and tear at bay, thus preserving the condition and optimal safety operation of the car.

You need to have your identification, registration and insurance cards, and a small amount of money with you when you drive. If you have a cell phone, carry it with you fully charged. Along with your first-aid emergency equipment, your vehicle should also carry the following items:

- Tire-changing equipment/spare tire (properly inflated)
- Rags, paper towels
- Window cleaner
- Jumper cables
- Can of tire inflator and sealant
- Motor oil, antifreeze, and brake fluid
- Container of water for radiator
- Sunglasses
- Plastic bags

Chapter 11

First Aid at Work

The work environment needs to be safe and healthy not only to avoid work-related illness and injury, but also so that you can perform your job properly while you are there. By ensuring your health and safety, your employer will have happier, healthier, and more productive employees. Work stress can also be harmful to your health and contribute to stress-related conditions such as insomnia and burnout. Learning how to cope with stress and deal with stress-related conditions can keep you healthier and safer at work, and can also help improve the overall quality of your life.

How Safe Is Your Workplace?

The Occupational Safety and Health Act of 1970 (OSH Act) was instituted by the U.S. Department of Labor to ensure safe and healthy work conditions for working men and women. This act grants the Occupational Safety and Health Administration (OSHA) the authority to impose and enforce standards or regulations affecting the safety and health of private-sector employees.

Every safety measure outlined for home safety also applies in the workplace for employee safety and for the safety of the public. In addition, employees need to be aware of and to practice fire, safety, health, and disaster protocols set up by employers. Workers need to know how to use and have access to such provisions as safe and ergonomic equipment and safety gear when called for, and need knowledge of proper body mechanics, knowledge of proper food handling, and good ventilation and lighting. A safe workplace needs to:

- Be free from any recognized hazards and constructed with safety in mind
- Make all safety devices and gear, and proper tools and equipment available as needed
- Prohibit alcohol and narcotics
- Ensure employees protection from chemicals and biological agents such as bodily fluids, mold and mildew, and those found in research labs
- Provide protection from animals or animal waste in animal-related workplaces
- Make sure employees are aware of and practicing proper body mechanics and exercises to avoid injury
- Provide ample time for meals and breaks
- Ensure employees are able to enter and leave the workplace safely
- Ensure employees protection from mental stressors such as workplace harassment, bullies, and physical threats and violence

Fire Safety at Work

Workplace protocol should include fire extinguishers that are readily accessible; working, manual fire-alarm pull boxes on the walls; emergency lights; exit doors; unobstructed sprinkler heads; and sprinkler-system risers. In case of fire, access to the front and rear of the building should be unobstructed at all times, including clear access to fire hydrants, automatic sprinkler connections, and sprinkler control valves. Your workplace should have designated smoking areas with safe, noncombustible receptacles to extinguish smoking materials. Brush and vegetation and all other combustibles need to be kept clear of the building. Your office or workplace should be equipped with permanent wiring, not extension cords and surge suppressors connected to all computers. Owners and management need to maintain all equipment up to code and ensure that all combustibles are stored away from heat sources. In the event of a fire, pull fire alarms, call 911, exit the building, and wait for the fire department to arrive.

Fact

According to the CDC, overall workplace injury and illness has declined in recent years, but the rate of fatal workplace injuries has increased. For this reason you need to understand and know how to administer emergency first aid, take all necessary workplace safety precautions, and have a clear understanding of your workplace emergency response policies.

Preventing Injuries in the Workplace

Back injuries, stress-related health problems, carpel-tunnel syndrome, headaches, and mental-health problems are all conditions that may result from poor ergonomic workplace conditions including temperature, station design, lighting, noise, rotating shifts, inadequate meals and breaks, and machine design. Small corrective measures can prevent large and costly problems. For example, using ergonomically correct chairs and keyboards, properly positioned workstations, a mouse with the correct tension, wrist supports, telephone neck supports, ample lighting, frequent breaks, and proper foot support are measures that will help prevent many physical problems.

Fact

Ergonomics is the science of refining the design of products to optimize them for human use, taking into consideration human characteristics such as height, weight, and proportions and including such information as human hearing, sight, and temperature preferences.

Carpal-Tunnel Syndrome

The emergence and ubiquity of computers in the workplace has contributed to an epidemic of repetitive stress injuries most commonly called carpal-tunnel syndrome. Carpal-tunnel syndrome is a painful, progressive condition caused by compression of a nerve in the wrist due to repetitive motion, improper positioning of the wrist, and repeated stressors such as the continual vibrations from using a jackhammer or even a sewing machine.

First Aid for Carpal-Tunnel Syndrome

The following measures can be used to avoid carpal-tunnel syndrome:

- Reducing your force and relaxing your grip by tapping keys softly
- Using a big pen with an oversized, soft grip and free-flowing ink
- Using a keyboard and mouse with the proper tension
- Keeping keyboards at elbow height or just slightly below, with the wrist at a relaxed middle position, not bent up or down
- Taking frequent breaks
- Practicing carpal-tunnel exercises before and after your work shift and during your breaks
- Alternating tasks if you can
- Improving your posture
- Keeping your hands warm

You may also wear splints at work and while sleeping if you have symptoms of carpal-tunnel syndrome such as tingling or numbness in fingers or hands; pain or weakness in wrists, arms, or hands; and loss of feeling in some fingers. While you sleep, the tendency is to keep the wrists flexed; wearing splints at night will keep your wrists from flexing. Wrist splints are available at most pharmacies and many retail outlets. Anyone with moderate to severe symptoms needs to see their doctor.

Following are some carpal-tunnel exercises you can try:

1. In a standing position, lift and extend both arms straight out. Flex your entire hand at the wrist as if saying stop. Hold in this position for five seconds.
2. Straighten your wrists and relax your fingers so that arms, wrists, hands, and fingers are level and fingers are pointing forward.
3. Maintain the level position while making a fist; clench it tightly and hold for five seconds.
4. With fists clenched, flex your wrists down and hold for five seconds.
5. Straighten your wrists and relax your fingers so that arms, wrists, hands, and fingers are level and fingers are pointing forward (as in position 2).
6. Repeat all of the steps ten times, followed by standing with your arms relaxed by your sides.

Back Injuries

Back injuries are one of the most common and costly work-related disorders in the United States. Lower-back pain is responsible for many days of lost work, increased number of workers-compensation claims, increased monetary business losses, and undue suffering every day. Many back injuries can be prevented by practicing measures for good back health including using ergonomically correct chairs and equipment, good posture, and regular exercise and conditioning. In addition, you should always practice good body mechanics and use proper lifting techniques (see following) to protect your spine and prevent back strain and injuries.

Proper lifting technique includes the following:

1. Always stand close to the weight or load in order to reduce excessive strain on your back muscles. Try to estimate which direction the load will move after lifting so that you can position your feet to allow for this movement without twisting the trunk of your body.
2. Place one foot firmly alongside the load to be lifted, and the other just behind the object with your heels flat, in order to have a wider, more stable base from which to lift.
3. Bend your knees and squat down. Keeping your back erect, grasp the load and use your leg muscles to lift the object.
4. Make sure to grip the load firmly from underneath. Use your entire hand rather than just your fingers. Keep your arms straight using your shoulder muscles to help lift the weight.
5. Stand and lift, straightening your legs gradually from a squatting to an erect position. Avoid jerking when you lift and setting down a load too quickly.
6. Carry the load close to your body, as near as you are able to your own center of balance, keeping your back erect.
7. Turning should only be done by using your whole frame, not just your trunk. Twisting places the load outside your center of balance and strains muscles not intended for lifting.

8. To lower the load; reverse the lifting operation. With your back straight, bend your legs at the knees to a squat position, place the load down, withdraw your hands from the object, and stand up using the same method as lifting a load, using your legs and keeping your back straight.

9. Only one person should give the directions for the team, whether it is two or more that are lifting and carrying a load. The load needs to be well balanced and distributed evenly.

10. When you need to raise a load to shoulder height or higher, lift it first to about waist height, then rest one end of it on a ledge; if necessary, shift the position of your hands to accomplish this and push the load straight up. Reverse the process when lowering objects.

11. Always keep your chin up while lifting, because your back is likely to be straighter and your ability to lift while avoiding back injury is greatly improved.

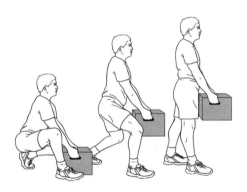

Proper lifting technique

First Aid for Back Pain

Stop any activity or exercise that increases your pain, and for the first few days take the following steps:

1. Take an OTC pain reliever.
2. Apply a covered cold pack to the area for five to ten minutes every hour during the first twenty-four to forty-eight hours.
3. For continued pain after two days, use a heating pad on the area.
4. Avoid bed rest; keep moving, but protect your back from strain and sudden jarring movements.
5. Seek medical care for intense pain or pain that continues for four to six weeks. Most incidents of back pain resolve in about one month.

 Essential

Injury prevention includes overall physical conditioning. Exercises that strengthen the abdomen are important and necessary in order to help prevent back injuries.

Stress and Personal Safety in the Workplace

A little pressure is requisite for performance, but excessive pressure can lead to unhealthy levels of stress. A little stress gives you the energy and motivation to meet challenges, goals, and deadlines at work. Stress pushes you to achieve so that you accomplish things that result in feelings of satisfaction and happiness. But too much stress has negative impacts, such as exhaustion, frustration, dissatisfaction, and even mental and physical health problems, and eventually total burn out.

Unrealistic demands in a job and insufficient control over job tasks and situations often lead to unhealthy amounts of stress. Job uncertainty, such as fear of lay-off and increased demands for overtime, are also typical negative stressors. Feeling pressured or having little encouragement and praise at work can also lead to stress, burnout, and decreased job satisfaction. An accumulation of stressors has the potential to create negative and unhealthy stress. Stressors can result from factors such as degree of responsibility, conflicting job demands, and working too much or too little, which can lead to boredom. Pace and variety of work, personal feelings about the meaningfulness of work, level of autonomy, or the ability to make decisions about your job and tasks are factors that may contribute to stress. Environmental factors such as noise, light, room temperature, and air quality may add to physical problems as well as emotional stress. Shift work and work hours that can lead to sleep deprivation are often stressors that can lead to burnout.

Dealing with Workplace Stress

Workplace stresses and degree of stress have a lot of variation, so strategies to reduce or prevent stress also have to be multifaceted. Environmental stressors like noise control, poor lighting, and ergonomics need to addressed, but it's up to you to report these stressors to your boss or management. If you feel you have too much responsibility and too little authority, are subject to unfair labor practices, or have an inadequate, undefined job description, you can address concerns by talking with your supervisors first and then your union or other organizations or grievance or personnel offices. Ask to have your job description clarified, and don't stay in a job that you hate and don't think you'll ever feel differently about.

The old expression, "Find a job you love and you'll never work another day in your life," holds true. And while it may not be possible to change jobs, you can approach your supervisor with all of your concerns and about providing stress-management training; and you can take advantage of your employee-assistance program (EAP) if available; this will improve your ability to cope with difficult work situations. In order to keep stress at bay, practice the following stress-reduction techniques in your daily life:

1. Get an adequate amount of sleep (make sleep a priority).
2. Develop a support system to share your feelings and get validation and support.
3. Maintain a regular exercise program.
4. Eat a nutritious and balanced diet.
5. Reduce or eliminate caffeine and sugar.
6. Don't use alcohol or drugs to self-medicate.
7. Set aside some "Me" time every day.

Beyond Stress

Burnout is a state of extreme emotional and physical exhaustion caused by prolonged and excessive stress over time. It may occur after feeling overwhelmed and unable to meet continual and constant demands. As the stressors continue, a person will begin to lose any interest or motivation that first brought them to pursue their job or take on their current role. Burnout reduces productivity radically, causes feelings of fatigue and apathy, and increasingly powerless, hopeless, cynical, and resentful.

Burnout can eventually threaten your job, your health, and your relationships. You are usually aware of being under a lot of stress, but you may not always notice burnout when it happens. Burnout's roots are in excessive stress, and it's a gradual process, so learn to recognize symptoms and address them early on. Signs and symptoms of burnout include:

- Feelings of frustration and powerlessness
- Hopelessness
- Being emotionally drained
- Detachment, isolation, and withdrawal (both at work and at home)
- Feeling trapped
- Feelings of failure
- Irritability
- Sadness
- Cynicism

Many of the stress-prevention techniques outlined previously can also help prevent burnout. But the best way to head off job burnout is to change what you are doing, whether that means changing careers or jobs in your workplace. If neither of these is an option for you, there are still a number of steps you can take to recover from burnout, including talking to your employer about clarifying your job description. You may be unrealistically overextended or doing work you didn't sign on for and are not getting paid for. Request a transfer to another department, or ask for new or more varied duties.

Alert!

By law, you have the right to feel comfortable, stay safe, and be treated fairly at work, including being protected from feeling personally threatened. Contact the U.S. Department of Labor Occupational Safety and Health Administration (OSHA) office to report accidents, unsafe working conditions, or health and safety violations. Their toll-free number is 1-800-321-OSHA (6742).

Where Is Your Emergency Station?

Any workplace that involves potential eye injuries such as working with corrosive, irritating, toxic, or tissue-damaging materials needs to be equipped with an emergency eye-wash station to protect you from serious eye damage or blindness. Workplaces that have potential chemical, biological, or radiological hazards need to be equipped with emergency shower stations. All other workplaces need to have a central emergency location where emergency supplies are located. The station or area should include the following:

- Emergency phone numbers
- The location of a fire-alarm manual pull-station posted
- Two portable fire extinguishers
- First-aid supplies
- Flashlights and batteries
- Approved power strips and extension cords
- A portable AM/FM radio with batteries and emergency radio or walkie-talkie
- A laboratory spill kit if needed

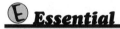

Essential

All workers need to be educated about any onsite hazards such as flammable materials, toxic chemicals, radioactive sources, or water-reactive substances. Also, someone needs to be the designated "in charge" person during work hours.

Your workplace first-aid kit should have the essential items outlined in Chapter 1 in quantities sufficient for the numbers of people employed, as well as the following items:

- 1 or more large, absorbent compresses
- 16 or more 1" × 3" adhesive bandages
- Several rolls of adhesive tape
- Smelling salts or ammonia inhalants
- 10 or more packets of povidone-iodine
- A dozen pairs of medical-exam gloves (latex and nonlatex)
- 4 or more sterile pads

- 1 large triangular bandage
- 1 eye patch
- 1 ounce of eye wash
- 1 chemical cold pack
- 2"-wide roller bandages
- 3"-wide roller bandages
- CPR barrier device

Where Is Your AED?

Learning to use the AED should also be a part of your emergency protocol, planning, and training. According to OSHA, cardiac arrest causes 15 percent of workplace fatalities, and 40 percent of these lives could be saved with the use of an AED within five minutes of arrest. Having an AED that can be reached in two or three minutes by every location of your workplace is a matter of life and death.

CPR rescue attempts that use an AED improve survival rates by as much as 49 percent, according to the American Heart Association. That's why it's critical to have access to an AED particularly in locations with large population groups and in homes where family members have serious health problems particularly heart disease.

Keeping Your Own Emergency Kit

While your workplace has a comprehensive first-aid kit, it is not going to be personalized for your individual needs. That's why it's a good idea to have your own small kit, containing items that you typically use, including any over-the-counter medications that you use regularly and a small store of your regular medications. As well as a basic first-aid kit, it's a good plan to keep a pair of comfortable walking shoes at your workplace in case of any evacuation, or even a planned drill—you may find yourself having to walk a long distance in shoes that are not designed for walking. Keep some bottled water and snacks at your workstation, along with a flashlight and extra batteries. Always bring some cash and coins, and even keep extra clothing at work (warm clothes in the winter) in case of accidents.

Calling 911 from Work

Any time you have a serious emergency requiring emergency response at work, you should call 911. See Chapter 1 for more information on when to call 911. In addition, you should call 911 if you or your coworkers have any doubts or concerns, even if you aren't sure the dispatcher knows how to help. When calling 911 from work, you need to remember to dial any prefixes necessary to obtain an outside line before dialing 911. In most 911 calls, a computer in the dispatch center shows the number and address of the phone you're using, but at a workplace the location of the main switchboard may be the only location appearing on the dispatcher's computer, so it's important that you provide accurate directions.

Chapter 12

Vacation Safety

During the year, you dream and plan about how you are going to spend your vacation time: traveling, going to the beach or the mountains, or just short weekend trips. When your vacation time finally arrives, make sure to keep it relaxed and fun, with the same awareness and planning for safety that you practice in your day-to-day life. In fact, you need to be even more aware when you're relaxing in unfamiliar places and locations. Planning for a fun and enjoyable vacation understandably takes first priority, but before you leave, take the necessary steps and precautions to make your vacation a safe one as well.

What to Pack

You don't want to end up paying $4 or more for a single bandage or pack of acetaminophen at the concierge desk, or even worse, have to do without, so take care in planning your vacation kit. Your vacation first-aid kit should include the same items as the kit you have at home, plus the following:

- A chemical cold pack or two for treating bruises and sprains
- Suntan lotion (SPF 15–SPF 30 is recommended)

- Bismuth subsalicylate for traveler's diarrhea
- Moleskin for blisters
- Lip balm
- Moist towelettes for cleaning hands
- Hand sanitizer
- OTC medications for nausea
- Water-purification tablets
- Insect repellent
- Elastic bandages for support or swelling
- Topical pain reliever
- Zip-top freezer bags
- Insect-sting relief pads
- Sanitary napkins (they are sterile and great for compresses to stop bleeding)
- Butterfly bandages
- A copy of your family medical history
- A list or chart including phone numbers of pediatricians and family doctors
- Any prescription medications you are taking in the original bottles; or, if you are using traveler's containers, be sure to record dosages and exact names of each drug
- First-aid manual
- Guidebook
- A phrase book that covers vocabulary on illnesses and talking to a doctor

Some people also like to take such things as cold medicine, a nasal decongestant, zinc lozenges, vitamin C and echinacea, and a can opener and bottle opener.

A great container for your traveling first-aid kit could be a small cooler with a zipper and shoulder strap. They have the ability to keep items at an even temperature, are lightweight and easy to fit in with other luggage, and easy to carry.

 Essential

Make sure to bring your doctor's phone number and the number of any recommended specialists in travel medicine in case you need a consultation or a second opinion while traveling. Keep these numbers handy and make sure that everyone traveling with you knows where to find them.

Sunglasses are a must for sunny destinations, but make sure to avoid yellow- or blue-lens sunglasses because they tend to distort colors and are not safe choices for driving. Sunglasses should block 99–100 percent of UVA and UVB rays according to the American Academy of Ophthalmology, so make sure to check the label when you purchase a pair—it should tell you the amount of protection the sunglasses provide.

What to Ask Before You Go

Now that global travel is on the increase, there are more health and safety considerations than ever before. The CDC has developed what they call The Yellow Book that provides comprehensive and current information on health recommendations and immunization requirements for international travelers. To search their tips and requirements for healthy travel, just go to *www.cdc.gov* and search for The Yellow Book. The CDC also has comprehensive health information that applies to all travel destinations. It's vital to know which illnesses may be encountered in each country so as to get all the vaccinations you or those traveling with you may need.

 Fact

The International Association for Medical Assistance to Travelers (IAMAT) is a nonprofit organization that offers phone assistance at 1-716-754-4883 and can be e-mailed at *iamat@sentex.net* for any health or medical travel-related questions or information.

If you or anyone in your party has altered immunocompetence due to illnesses such as HIV or diabetes, you may need the advice of your doctor before you travel. Special considerations are also important if you are pregnant or breastfeeding, or traveling with infants or children. That's why it's important to schedule a visit to your doctor or even a travel-medicine provider.

Vaccinations and Other Health Considerations

You may be able to obtain necessary immunizations at your state and local health departments. If your local departments don't have travel clinics, they are usually able to provide referrals for the area that takes care of vaccines for travelers. In addition, the doctor, department, or travel clinic you go to will be able to answer your questions about food and water safety, avoiding insects, and more. Depending on where you'll be visiting, you should know and understand a variety of illnesses related to that country.

Generally, vaccines need time to become effective in your body, and some need to be given in a series administered over a period of days to weeks. Get the information you need and start on any necessary vaccinations at least four to six weeks before your trip. Depending on your health, age, and vacation destination, you also may need shots, medications, and other information about how to protect your health while traveling, so see your doctor at least a month ahead of time, even if you are not going to be globetrotting.

Questions about Food and Water Safety

Another important consideration is the potential for infections such as *Escherichia coli* (E. coli), bacillary dysentery, hepatitis A, and other less common infectious diseases such as parasites from consuming contaminated food or drink while traveling. It's also possible to contract respiratory, neurological, and diarrhea diseases as well as ear, eye, and skin infections from inadvertent ingestion of water while swimming or diving in lakes, rivers, oceans, and improperly or inadequately treated swimming pools.

Find out if your destination is lacking chlorinated tap water or if hygiene and sanitation are inadequate. When traveling to destinations with potentially contaminated food and water, you should plan to only drink beverages like tea and coffee that are made with boiled water, bottled beverages and water, carbonated mineral water, soft drinks, beer, and wine and make sure to never consume ice, as it could also be contaminated. In this case, you also need to avoid milk and milk products such as cheese, salads, and all uncooked vegetables, and to be safe, eat only cooked food that is still hot (never reheat cold food) and fruit that you personally wash in clean water and peel yourself. It's also necessary and wise to brush your teeth with bottled water.

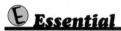 **Essential**

Avoid swallowing water during aquatic activities, even in pools in the United States. All water even in swimming pools may not be properly or adequately treated and may contain germs that can potentially make you sick if swallowed.

Traveler's Health Insurance

Most health-insurance plans, Medicare, or Medicaid won't provide coverage for any health or medical care received outside of the United States. That's why you should consider asking your travel agent about travel insurance in case you or someone in your family needs medical care while away. Depending on your type of travel, whether you are visiting a developing country or going on a safari, you need to find out what policy is going to give you adequate coverage. Ask about features like twenty-four-hour, toll-free, English-language phone assistance and plans that provide immediate and direct payment to the medical-care provider.

What to Ask When You Get There

When you get to your destination outside of the United States, find out where the U.S. embassy or consulate is located and how to get there, as they can help you find necessary medical care. Also get directions to the nearest hospital or clinic. Consult with your guidebook, hotel, or tourist office for recommendations on local doctors. In remote areas, you may have to rely on a police station, military base, or missionary post to give you help and information. Ask how and where you can make international calls and access the Internet at your vacation destination. Check out the area and locations of the closest grocery store where you can buy bottled water and other safe, packaged food and beverages. Remember to never eat food from street vendors. In foreign countries where there are concerns about clean water, it's important to remember to wash wounds only with bottled water.

Diarrhea in Foreign Countries

The infamous Delhi-belly diarrhea may end your vacation or it may end up being mild and stay that way—if you take measures to avoid solid foods until the diarrhea goes away and rehydrate yourself with clean, bottled water. The World Health Organization (WHO) has formulated rehydration salts to treat diarrhea. You can buy packets of these salts at stores and pharmacies in most developing countries.

First Aid for Diarrhea

Most cases of diarrhea are self-limiting; that is, they run a short course and resolve on their own. Eating yogurt can help prevent diarrhea because it introduces helpful enzymes into your GI tract. Nonprescription medications such as Bismuth subsalicylate may help treat diarrhea in adults only if you do not have other signs of illness, such as fever, abdominal cramping or discomfort, or bloody stools. If you do get diarrhea, adults and children over two years of age should take the following steps.

1. Let your stomach rest and avoid food for several hours or until you feel better.
2. Rehydrate by taking frequent, small sips of bottled or boiled water or a rehydration drink, and eating small bites of salty crackers.
3. If you have WHO rehydration salts, add one packet to bottled or treated water, using the proper amounts of salts and water as directed on the package.
4. Follow a simple diet of bland foods, such as bread, potatoes, bananas, crackers, and rice.
5. Resume a regular diet when your diarrhea is gone.

In children two years old or younger, continue to breastfeed or bottlefeed as normal, don't restrict food, and use WHO rehydration salts along with food as long as diarrhea continues.

Seek medical attention immediately for anyone with fever or persistent vomiting, if there is blood or pus in the stool, or if the diarrhea continues for more than forty-eight hours, because antibiotics may be needed.

 Essential

In order to avoid becoming dehydrated and to stay healthy, make sure to drink at least two quarts of water a day, or at least one quart of water for every fifty pounds of body weight, while traveling.

Staying in a Hotel Room

When you arrive at your hotel, find out where the nearest safety exists are and plan your own safety escape. Ask at the desk how they want to be informed in case of an emergency, if they have emergency protocol, and how to use the phone for emergencies.

Keep fire safety in mind while staying in a hotel. It's not a good idea to use candles, matches, and lighters, and never dry clothing on heaters, a fireplace, or woodstove in your hotel room. In case of fire or if you hear a fire alarm, leave the hotel using the nearest fire-exit stairway and do not take time to collect any of your belongings. As in any fire situation, feel the door for heat and check for smoke before opening it. If you feel heat on the door or see smoke, look around for a different way to leave.

Bedbugs

Bedbugs are tiny, flat bugs smaller than an apple seed. They live all over the world in every country and are found everywhere from youth hostels to five-star hotels. Bedbugs travel in suitcases and live in beds, carpets, behind baseboards, under wallpaper, and in small cracks and crevices throughout a room. There are a couple of ways to identify bedbugs in your hotel room. First, they tend to leave tiny reddish or black streaks on sheets. Second, they leave small, itchy bumps that you may find upon waking in the morning, often in linear groups of three commonly referred to as "breakfast, lunch, and dinner."

If you suspect you have been bitten or see telltale signs of bedbugs, grab your suitcases and head to the desk to ask for a new room. Also, be sure to shake out your suitcases to rid them of any stowaways. You can then treat any bites with 1% hydrocortisone or antihistamine cream for the itch and inflammation.

Childproofing Your Hotel Room

If you have children, then you need to childproof your hotel room. Your hotel may offer a childproofing kit, so inquire when you get there. Pay attention to things like blinds and loose or dangling cords. Watch your children around any electrical outlets, furniture with sharp corners, or loose equipment. Move furniture away from any windows if you can. Talk to your children about never standing on chairs or jumping from bed to bed, and don't let them on the balconies alone. Like all home-safety measures, you need to keep soaps, shampoos, plastic bags, matches, and toiletries out of the reach of children. Take special precautions about such things as dry-cleaning bags, glasses, coffeemakers, and hairdryers. Always carefully check the hot water for the bath to make sure the water is not too hot. Make sure that any alcohol in the mini fridge is out of reach of young children, including partially empty glasses.

Children can suffer head injuries, crushed nerves, internal injuries, and broken bones from pulling TV sets on top of themselves. In many cases, these accidents happen because televisions are set on top of a simple stand or cart, although children have pulled them from wall units, shelving, and from atop dressers as well. Make sure that the television in your room is secured to the dresser or table. Instruct your children not to climb, play with, or pull on the television or the stand, and not to play with cords, plugs, and television buttons.

Most experts don't recommend sleeping with a baby in an adult bed, because there is a danger that the baby will slip between the bed and the wall or under a pillow or blanket. Call ahead to find out what kind of crib the hotel offers so that you can bring your own portable folding bed if necessary. These infant beds are made to nestle in between your pillows at the top of your bed and will keep your infant safe.

When traveling with babies, make sure that you get a room with a crib and double check that the crib is set up securely and properly and that the mattress is firmly supported and fits snugly. Just as at home, the sheets need to fit the mattress securely and the crib needs to stay clutter free. A crib should be manufactured after 1986 in the United States to meet safety regulations. Exercise caution when using a crib provided by a hotel, because many hotels have outdated and recalled products, including cribs.

Staying in a Tent

When you go camping, be prepared to care for any cuts, scrapes, and scratches by bringing a well-stocked first-aid kit, your first-aid manual, and all the comforts that you desire. Roughing it usually means campfires, so be sure to bring along some saline solution to wash irritated eyes if you get ashes or cinders in them while sitting too close to the fire. Cotton swabs are great for applying lotion to bug bites, rashes, and scratches, and tweezers are a must for removing splinters and thorns. An aloe-vera solution for skin irritations, lip balm for the lips, zinc oxide for sun and skin protection, burn cream, a flashlight with spare batteries, a whistle for each camper, sanitary napkins to control bleeding, and if needed, a snakebite kit, are all must-have camping first-aid items.

A good tent should have a built-in sheet underneath to prevent cold (and insects) from getting inside, and another separate sheet to put underneath the tent. You should also bring all the appropriate clothing and gear you need to stay warm and safe. In addition, while enjoying camping and other outdoor activities, it's critical to drink at least two quarts of water a day, or at least one quart of water for every fifty pounds of body weight, and more with any vigorous activity to avoid dehydration. Avoid dehydrating high-protein foods and caffeinated beverages. If you notice your urine is becoming a darker yellow, you also need to increase fluid intake.

More Advice Concerning the Great Outdoors

Always appoint an experienced person to watch the group for signs of injury, fatigue, hypothermia, dehydration, sunstroke, frostbite, or any other illness. Avoid hypothermia by staying rested, maintaining good nutrition, and consuming lots of high-energy food. In addition, bring and use the proper clothing for the area and the time of year. If you become tired, injured, or lost, make camp early. If you have any signs of hypothermia, discuss it with your group and take immediate action together.

 Essential

Don't forget! As soon as you stop, you run a greater risk of hypothermia, so weigh the dangers of treating an injury with rest against the potential for hypothermia. The danger of exposure may be the greater risk.

To avoid frostbite, bring and wear the proper clothing for the area and for the weather; maintain good nutrition; drink water; maintain core temperature by staying active; and use your buddies to create a system to check critical areas such as face, nose, and ears. Don't wait for crisis; respond with immediate treatment for all symptoms, no matter how minor they seem.

Fact

Make sure to have a method for calling for help, an understanding of first aid, and first-aid supplies whenever traveling. And be aware that accidents are most common when vacations involve traveling on the road, to beaches, staying in hotels, skiing, and in remote locations.

Let Common Sense Be Your Guide

In any unknown territory, it's essential to take extra precautions to avoid danger and prevent accidents. It's also best to plan for the very worst scenarios. For these types of trips, you must pack a survival kit that includes not only your first-aid kit, but a good and comprehensive map; a compass; at least two flashlights with spare batteries; a waterproof fire starter; a good, versatile hunting knife; personal shelter; whistles; warm clothing; sturdy, comfortable hiking boots; rain gear; high-energy food; and water. Take a first-aid manual, and if you are able, take a course before you leave to learn about and have hands-on practice with the ABCs of first aid and how to treat and manage emergencies. Use your senses and your common sense and stay away from dangerous areas where hazards of nature may occur, such as rock falls, floods, rip currents, rapids, avalanches, hazardous plants and animals, any other hazardous terrain, areas of poor sanitation, and treacherous climates.

Everyone in your group needs to know the locations of the first-aid kit, who their buddy is, and the overall supervisor and camp leader who needs to set the pace based on the slowest individual. Before you leave for any outdoor trip, you need to inform at least one friend at home what your plans are, when you are expected home, when you are expected at certain checkpoints, and other clues that may indicate your need for rescue. If an accident or injury occurs, make sure that everyone stays calm. Even in the case of becoming lost or separated from your group, stay calm and see if you are able to retrace your steps. Know how to use your compass, identify points, and use your common sense. Chances are, while roughing it, you may not be near any help or a hospital, so on all outdoor trips it's critical to be careful, vigilant, prepared, and safe.

Chapter 13

Other Safety Concerns

According to a 2006 survey by the Anxiety Disorders Association of America, almost all working Americans suffer anxiety or stress from daily living. This hurried and pressured culture contributed to physical, mental, and emotional conditions and increased use and abuse of prescription medications such as tranquilizers, antidepressants, and anti-anxiety medications. It also affects abuse of over-the-counter medications for the production of methamphetamines and Robbotripping (abuse of cold medicine to get high), as well as rises in alcoholism, obesity, suicide, drug addiction, cigarette addiction, and other harmful behaviors.

Depression Signs to Look For

Depression is much more common in adults, although it does occur in children and teens as well. Because children have different behaviors than adults, their symptoms of depression are also different. While a depressed adult may seem sad or may cry, children are more likely to act out and behave badly or have out-of-proportion and inappropriate anger. They may have a decreased interest in activities they normally enjoy, become pickier about food, and be irritable. Most people will have bouts of sadness or feel low from time to time and lasting for a few days, but this is not the same as major depression. A person with major depression will have at least five of the following symptoms persistently for at least two weeks:

- Sadness, depressed mood, crying
- Irritability, lack of satisfaction in accomplishments
- Easy frustration, lack of follow through
- Poor self-esteem, low motivation, and reluctance to accept new projects
- Decreased interest in activities that were previously pleasurable
- Changes in appetite; rapid weight gain or loss
- Changes in sleep patterns; sleeping too much or too little
- Slowed body movements; slow, soft speech
- Fatigue, lack of energy
- Poor concentration, attention, and memory
- Thoughts or expressions of death or suicide

Another type of depression is manic depression, or bipolar disorder, that alternates with symptoms of depression and those of being "wired" and exhibiting reckless behavior such as shoplifting or gambling. When in a manic or wired state, a person may tend to be grandiose, not sleep, exhibit careless sexual activity, talk nonstop, and be rebellious or irritable.

Fact

According to the National Alliance on Mental Illness (NAMI), major depression is the most commonly diagnosed mental disorder, is a serious and often debilitating illness, and affects close to seventeen million Americans.

Talk about Problems

Everyone gets sad and blue sometimes, but if you, your loved one, or your child are having problems related to grades or school attendance, relationships, alcohol, drugs, or sex, or are exhibiting uncontrolled behavior, the problem may be a depression that can be helped with treatment. Depression that isn't treated may end up getting worse and last longer. Talk to the person you love and tell them that depression, or problems with substance abuse, doesn't mean that they are weak, or a failure, or not trying hard enough. It means they have a real medical illness and need treatment, usually talk therapy, medicine, or both together. Be sure to emphasize that most people who seek treatment for depression start to feel better in just a few weeks. Let the person with a substance-abuse problem know that they have your support, and encourage them to get the professional help that they need. Assure the person that they are not alone, and that there are many people who can help, such as professionals at mental-health centers, the family doctor, someone in the clergy, or a school counselor or nurse.

Suicide

Suicide is a multifaceted problem with many causes, but there are usually warning signs such as depression and substance abuse. The vast majority of suicidal people will give a sign of their intent: some may talk about suicide, call suicide crisis lines, or threaten suicide. Warning signs of suicide include:

- Suicidal ideation (suicidal thoughts or actions)
- Excessive, increased substance abuse
- Expressing or feeling that there is no reason to live
- Anxiety (agitation or insomnia)
- Feeling trapped
- Feeling hopeless
- Withdrawal from friends, family, or society
- Anger
- Recklessness
- Dramatic mood changes
- Personality changes such as strange or unusual behavior
- Decreased interest in things they used to enjoy
- Changes in eating or sleeping habits
- Withdrawal from friends and family
- Increased absences and decreased performance at school or work
- Changes in personal hygiene habits
- Exhibiting a strong sense of guilt, shame, or emptiness
- An obsession with death
- Giving away personal and prized belongings, including pets

Teen Suicide

According to the CDC, teen suicide is the third lead-ing cause of death among teenagers in the United States and has become a critical problem. Nearly 2,000 teens commit suicide every year in the United States. In a school auditorium holding 100 students, statistics show that at least twenty of them have had serious thoughts of suicide and at least eight of them have attempted suicide. Female youths attempt suicide more often than males, but the incidence of actual suicides is four times higher in male teens. Over 60 percent of teens use a gun to commit sui-cide and the majority of gun-related attempts or suicides with guns occur in the home. That's why it is vital to keep guns away from children of any age.

Depression, alcohol, and substance abuse are factors in 90 percent of teen suicides according to the *Journal of Clinical Psychiatry*. Because many teen suicides occur in families that have had a family member who has also attempted or committed suicide, it's believed that some disorders such as depression have genetic components. The following events can also influence teen suicide:

- Stress from fighting with friends
- Breaking up with girlfriends or boyfriends
- Getting into trouble at school or with the police
- Substance abuse
- Depression
- A history of physical or sexual abuse
- Poor communication with parents
- Incarceration for any reason

Teens are also influenced by hearing, seeing, and reading about other teen attempts and suicides, so all of these events need careful attention, discussion, and any necessary treatment.

First Aid for Suicide Attempts and Self-Harm

If you come across someone who has attempted suicide, or suspect an attempt, take note of whether the person may be under the influence of a drug, such as exhibiting slurred speech and lethargy, or self-inflicted injuries. Take the following steps; stay safe and away from any scenes with guns, weapons, or extremely violent behavior; and use universal precautions if you are able:

- In the case of a hanging, get the person down as quickly as possible.
- Call 911, check for breathing, and start CPR and other first-aid measures for injuries.
- Look for pills, look at the date of any prescriptions, and note the number of pills left and type of medication so that you can report to EMS.
- Look for a note to bring to the hospital or to give to EMS.
- Don't disturb the scene; in the event of death there will be a death-scene evaluation.
- Refrain from any judgmental remarks.

If the person is conscious, calm them, explaining that you are getting help and someone to talk to and they don't have to be afraid, while you administer any necessary first aid and wait for help to arrive.

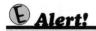

Alert!

> If your teen has attempted suicide, statistics show that there is a greater chance he will make another attempt, so it's critical to understand and be aware of risk factors and signs and symptoms and to seek help for your child.

Preventing Suicide

If you are able to talk with the person frankly, listen closely, allow as much time as necessary, don't minimize the person's feelings, and do not offer any judgments. Talking about suicide decreases the probability that the person will act on their suicidal feelings. Include the following points in any discussion about suicide:

- Ask the person frankly if they are considering suicide. If the answer is yes, ask if they have a plan to commit suicide, and if so, how and where they plan to carry it out.
- Express your concerns and fears, but do not minimize or judge their feelings.
- Ask what you can do, and talk about who might be able to help, such as family or close friends.
- Explain that there is also professional help available from community agencies and crisis centers, as well as counseling and treatment.
- Together, make a plan for the next few hours and days, including contacting any professionals, and if you are able, go with the person to get help.

- Keep an eye on the person and the situation, and give them support and praise for their courage and strength in opening up and seeking help.

Realize what your own limitations are, and involve others in helping, supporting, and protecting the person in danger.

If you or someone you know is contemplating suicide, talk to your family doctor, call the National Suicide Prevention Lifeline at 1-800-273-TALK (1-800-273-8255), or contact the National Youth Violence Prevention Resource Center at 1-866-SAFEYOUTH (1-866-723-3968), 1-866-620-4160 (TTY), or e-mail your questions to NYVPRC@safeyouth.org.

Talk to Your Kids about Suicide

All available data shows that talking to your children lowers the risk of suicide, and that talking to them about suicide does not put thoughts or ideas into their head. When you talk to them, you give them the message that suicide is never an option and that help is always available. Kids lack maturity, and they tend to make small things into huge, enormously emotional, consuming issues. Never minimize anything your child is going through emotionally, as this will only add to feelings of hopelessness and despair. Take all of your child's concerns seriously and be available and approachable to discuss and troubleshoot issues with them. When issues are too big for you, it may be time to turn to a counselor, coach, clergy member, or doctor.

Be direct in communication with your child. If you hear your child mention death or indicate wanting to die, you need to ask them pointedly, "I've heard you mention wanting to be dead. Are you having thoughts about trying to kill or harm yourself?" If you feel that your child is thinking about suicide, always and without any hesitation get help immediately. Call your doctor, who can refer you to the appropriate help—a psychologist or psychiatrist. Call your local hospital and speak to the department of psychiatry, who will also direct you to the right source for help. Local mental-health associations and county medical societies will also give you proper referrals.

Talk to Your Kids about Drugs

Children are told that drugs are dangerous, but family medicine cabinets are often full of prescription and over–the-counter medications. Music, TV, movies, and other media make drug and alcohol use look acceptable and even desirable. Everything about drugs is confusing to children and teens today. It's your role as an adult to give your kids the facts about drugs.

Start talking to your kids early; at age six or seven, a child is able to understand concepts of staying healthy. Continue to answer any questions with short simple comments that are factual, not preachy. Increase the amount of information as children get older, and never stop telling your kids that drugs, cigarettes, and alcohol are harmful. Kids don't understand concepts well unless they are reinforced over and over, and with the constant barrage of media and other input they receive, you need to counter those messages with the truth and with facts—that drugs and alcohol can hurt your body, make you sick, and sometimes even kill you. Emphasize that you don't want them to have the problems that come with experimenting with things that will keep them from having a happy, successful, and healthy life.

 Fact

Start talking to your kids when they are very young, because studies show that many kids first try alcohol at age eleven, and marijuana as young as age twelve. Student surveys also show that when parents are available to listen, their kids are more likely to talk openly and to stay drug free.

Be a good example for your kids by not indulging in things that you are telling your kids not to do. Kids learn by your example. So if you need to take medication, do it when children are not present. Remember, they are following your lead.

Chapter 14

Emergency Preparedness

Some emergencies are disasters that have the potential to damage your home, the function of your community and economy, and the environment, as well as injuring a vast number of people. This chapter will focus on management of emergencies such as HAZMAT spills (any harmful liquid, solid, or gas), earthquakes, floods, tornadoes, hurricanes, meltdowns, and events related to terrorist attacks. You may be prepared for emergencies that involve your family, but you also need to be prepared for emergencies that may affect your home, the area you live in, your entire community, or even beyond.

An Overview of Emergency Preparedness

Imagine losing everything you own and everything you would need to know to start over from scratch; that is the information you will need to gather to begin your emergency preparedness plan. Also imagine you or a family member ending up in an unknown emergency room in an unknown condition, and with the limited information they can obtain, emergency workers are not sure they are giving the appropriate care. This is additional vital information you need to gather for your disaster records. There are myriad scenarios for many types of disasters, and overall emergency preparedness, or preparing for the worst, will help ensure the health, safety, and support of all your family members during any sudden disaster. By planning and preparing, you will be ready for disasters ranging from the need for sudden evacuation to events that may cause your family to be cut off from the outside world.

Gathering Information

Gathering information is an important and vital part of disaster preparedness. You will need to get together originals or copies of family records (birth, marriage, and death certificates); an inventory of valuable household goods; important telephone numbers; and copies of medical information, bank account numbers, and homeowner's and insurance policies. Start by creating a form for each family member that is small enough and convenient enough to carry on their person. The form should contain the following information for each person:

- Name
- Age
- Address
- Home and cell numbers
- Name of primary physician
- Allergies
- Prescription drugs and doses
- Past medical history
- Chronic conditions
- Emergency contacts, including nearby relatives or friends and an out-of-town and out-of-state relative

or friend (during regional emergencies, you may not be able to call locally, but you may often call long distance).

The U.S. Department of Homeland Security provides Americans with free preparedness information and easy-to-fill-out information forms at *www.ready.gov*. You may also get information by calling their toll-free number, 1-800-BE-READY.

Once you fill out an emergency-contact form for each member of your immediate family, you need to decide the best place to put the information so that it remains safe until you need it. To begin, print out or make a few copies of each list, have them laminated to protect them from water damage, and pick a central place to keep one copy and other locations in the house to store remaining copies.

Emergency responders usually look for information in the kitchen, and since in a natural disaster the refrigerator is usually left standing, keeping a sealed plastic container or a plastic zipper bag in the freezer might be the best place. Include information that emergency personnel may need to know for your children's health and safety in their school records, with caregivers, and at day care. Copies of all medical information should also be given to nearby relatives or close friends who may be called when you can't be found.

Other places to record information are on your computer, PDA, or other hand-held device. Make sure to also e-mail the information to yourself so that you can recover it from any computer should you be unable to access your own computer.

Have a Family Plan

Your local American Red Cross, emergency management, or civil-defense office can tell you what type of disasters have the potential to happen in your area and direct you toward necessary training such as CPR and first aid. They can also tell you what methods will be used for warning and informing the public of disasters, such as radio and TV, and how to be prepared. The local fire department can advise you about fire hazards in the home, and how to deal with fire situations during disasters.

Family and Neighborhood Meetings

Hold a family meeting to discuss disaster scenarios and what to do in case of evacuations or separation of family members. Explain your plans and preparations, and practice your plan. In case your family members are separated by disaster, decide on two different meeting places at a safe but accessible distance from your home, and somewhere in your neighborhood area in case you are not able to return home. Always take care to consider any special needs of disabled or sick and elderly persons, and plan for child care in case parents are injured or missing.

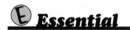
Essential

> Determine an out-of-state contact for everyone to call as a check-in point. Include your neighbors so the entire neighborhood will be prepared to work together using individual skills and resources.

Should You Stay or Should You Go?

Your state and local governments have established emergency plans for disasters both natural and man-made, specific to your area. Depending on your community, the methods of alerting you may differ, but a common method is to broadcast via emergency radio and TV broadcasts. You may also hear a special siren, receive telephone calls, or emergency workers may come to your door. During disasters or imminent disasters, it is vital to keep a TV or radio on to hear updates and instructions from local authorities and government officials. Keep an NOA Weather Radio on in your home to wake you up and alert you to weather alerts. Whatever the disaster or emergency, if firefighters, law enforcement, or local authorities recommend evacuation, you need to leave immediately.

In the case of hurricanes, you may have to make the decision whether you can ride out the storm in safety or if you need to evacuate. Generally, if your house is on the coastline or offshore islands, near a river, or in a flood plain, you should plan on evacuation. But if you live on higher ground and are not near any coastal lines, you may consider staying put. Be prepared by June when the hurricane season begins, so that you can have the information you need to evaluate the situation and make the best decision, whether to stay or leave.

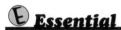

Essential

During times of imminent disasters, prepare ahead of time by having at least a half tank of gas in your vehicle, and while driving, keep your car windows closed and the air conditioner or heater off.

Find out the storm-surge history and elevation of your area, the safe routes to drive inland, and where official shelters are located. Listen to official bulletins on radio, TV, or NOAA Weather Radio, and stay tuned when a hurricane warning is issued for your area. If you decide to evacuate, drive safely and carefully by way of recommended evacuation routes to the nearest designated shelter.

If a flood warning is issued, you may be directed by authorities to leave if you are located in an area with potential for rising waters or in low-lying areas. If you are allowed to stay in your home, continue to listen to radio and television for updates. You also need to continue to prepare to evacuate should your home become damaged, or conditions change and you are told to leave by emergency personnel.

In the case of wildfire, the smoke may be so severe that the health risks outweigh any possible benefits of staying in your home. Smoke from fires may irritate your eyes, and respiratory system, and worsen chronic lung and heart diseases. Or the fire may begin to encroach on your home, jeopardizing your safety and causing you to evacuate. If you decide or are instructed to evacuate, listen to and follow directions about where to go, such as shelter locations and the safest routes to take.

Shelter-in-Place

You may also be given instructions in an emergency that involves HAZMAT, or chemical, biological, or radiological contaminants that are released into the environment, accidentally or intentionally, to seek shelter-in-place to keep you safe and indoors. When officials instruct the public to seek shelter-in-place, they want it to be immediate, which means wherever you are, whether the event occurs when you are at home or at work, you should not leave or drive or go outside.

During a shelter-in-place event, you must select and take refuge in a small interior room that is above ground level with no, or few, windows. Some chemicals may seep and pool into basements even if the windows are closed, because they are heavier than air, which is why you want to choose an upper-story room during any sort of HAZMAT threat. Plan a room that has your home's land telephone line because cell phones may be damaged or the lines overwhelmed during an emergency. Remember, shelter-in-place does not require you to seal off your entire home or building, only the room where you have taken refuge.

To create a shelter-in-place at home, perform the following steps:

1. Close and lock all windows and doors to the exterior.
2. Turn off fans, heating, and air-conditioning systems.
3. Close your fireplace dampers.
4. When there is also danger of explosion, close curtains, window shades, and blinds.
5. Take your family disaster-supplies kit along with your radio, your pets, and their food and water supplies.
6. Using heavy plastic sheeting and duct tape, seal all cracks around any vents, windows, and the door.
7. Keep your radio or television on and stay inside until you are told by officials that it is safe or you are instructed to evacuate.

If you are at work, participate in closing the business and ask any clients, customers, or visitors in the building to stay in order to provide them with safety. Then do the following:

1. If it is safe to do, everyone in the building should make contact with their persons to contact in case of emergency, letting them know where they are and that they are safe.
2. Put all phones on call forward, telephone-answering systems, or other available services.
3. Record a voice mail saying that the business is closed and that all employees and other persons plan to

remain inside the building until they are instructed by authorities that it is safe to leave.

4. Close and lock all exterior doors, windows, and other exterior openings.

5. For any danger of explosions, close curtains, window shades, and blinds just as you would in your home shelter-in-place.

6. Fans and heating and air-conditioning systems should be turned off, sealed, or disabled by employees that understand the building's systems, particularly those systems that automatically vent and exchange inside air with outside air.

7. Everyone then needs to gather in the safe room, and shut and lock the doors.

8. Record the name of everyone in the room. Then call the designated emergency contact for your business to report the number of people in the room, their names, and whether they are an employee, customer, visitor, or client.

 Essential

Wherever you may be during a HAZMAT event, remember that shelter-in-place instructions are usually instituted for only a few hours, not days or weeks, so don't be alarmed about oxygen, food, and water running out.

If you are at school, the school needs to close and the school's emergency plan needs to be activated immediately, and all students, faculty, visitors, and staff need to come inside. Follow all previously stated shelter-in-place procedures. In addition, the following steps should be taken:

1. At least one land-line telephone that shows the school's listed number when calling from the school should be in the rooms used for shelter-in-place.
2. The school secretary or some other designated person needs to answer telephone inquiries from concerned parents.
3. There needs to be a provision for communication between all rooms where people are sheltering-in-place.
4. Students should be allowed to use their cell phones to contact parents and guardians.
5. Ideally, announcements should be made over the school-wide public-address system.
6. Change the school voice-mail message to indicate that the school is closed and the students and staff are staying inside until advised that it is safe to leave by authorities.

Use several rooms such as classrooms, any large storage or utility rooms, meeting rooms, and even gymnasiums that don't have exterior windows so that there will be no problems associated with overcrowding.

If you are in your vehicle and hear a shelter-in-place announcement:

1. If you are very close to home, work, or a public building, drive there immediately and go inside.
2. If you are unable to get to any building promptly and safely, pull over to the side of the road and park in the shade or under a bridge to keep the car's interior from becoming overheated.
3. Turn off the engine and close the windows and all vents.
4. If you are carrying duct tape in your emergency kit, use it to seal the heating and air-conditioning vents.

Stay updated by listening to the radio regularly, and do not leave until informed that it is safe. Follow all directions of law-enforcement officers about traffic that may be detoured and roads that may be closed, and the instructions of local officials regarding shelter, food, water, and clean-up methods during and after any disaster or emergency. It is their role to help you stay safe.

 Question?

How can I find out what disasters can happen in my community?
Be prepared ahead of time for any potential disasters. You can find all the information you need for disaster preparedness at *www.ready.gov*.

Security Considerations

Even though you may be prepared, your safety and the safety of your family is more secure when the entire community works together. You can become involved by contacting Citizen Corps, which can connect you to disaster volunteer groups that prepare communities to respond to any emergency situation, terrorism, and disasters of all kinds. You can participate in the Citizen Corps community by volunteering for local law-enforcement activities through the Volunteers in Police Service (VIPS) Program. The Community Emergency Response Team (CERT) Program also offers education and training to neighborhood watch groups, community organizations, faith communities, school staff, workplace employees, scouting organizations, and other groups for disaster preparedness and responses such as fire safety, light search and rescue, team organization, and disaster medical operations. You may then work to assist other neighborhoods or workplaces after an event when professional responders may not be immediately available. For questions about the CERT program or Citizen Corps, you may contact the National Office of Citizen Corps at *citizencorps@dhs.gov*.

What to Pack and Where to Keep It

During or after a disaster of any type, you may expect relief workers and officials to appear right away, but they may not be able to be there for everyone immediately. It may take hours or even days for you to get any help or relief, so packing to prepare for days without access to food and basic necessities is vital. Preparing for disasters before they hit will help ensure the health and safety of your family and your ability to cope with a multitude of disaster scenarios. Your family needs to be prepared for being confined to your home, and for any immediate evacuation.

Stocking Your Home

Absolute basics you need to stock your home with for disaster emergencies include the following:

- Water
- Food
- A first-aid kit that is only to be used for disaster emergencies, including prescription and nonprescription drugs, necessary tools and supplies, sanitation supplies, clothing and bedding, and important family documents
- Any specialty items for family members such as infants and elderly or disabled persons
- Entertainment items like books, videos, and games

Store items you will need during evacuation in a container such as a large camping backpack, covered and sealed trash bin, duffle bag, or any other containers that are easy to transport and carry. Store a minimum of a gallon a day of water for each person (enough for three days) in unbreakable containers, preferably plastic bottles. Each person needs to have two quarts to drink and two quarts for hygiene, sanitation, and food preparation. In hot climates, people need to store more water to compensate for increased loss of hydration from perspiration.

Fact

You need to store one gallon of water per person, per day, for at least three days for drinking and sanitation during disasters.

Each person also needs a supply of foods that are compact and lightweight and don't require cooking, refrigeration (nonperishable), or preparation, particularly using water. Include such things as the following:

- Canned meats, fruits, and vegetables
- Juices in unbreakable containers
- Salt, pepper, sugar, and spices
- High-energy foods and snacks such as dried fruits, crackers, granola bars, trail mix, and peanut butter and jelly
- Vitamins
- Cookies and wrapped hard candy
- Cereals
- Instant coffee and tea bags
- Infant formula and foods

You will need a first-aid kit for your home, and one for each car. Your kit should be a combination of the supplies you have in your standard kit outlined in Chapter 1 and the kit you would take traveling or camping outlined in Chapter 12. In a separate container, store the following essential tools and supplies:

- Emergency preparedness manual
- Fire extinguisher (small canister, ABC type)
- Flashlight
- Paper cups, plates, and plastic utensils or mess kits
- Manual can opener and utility knife
- Battery-operated radio
- Batteries
- Cash, change, or travelers checks
- One or more small, compact, emergency tube tents, that roll up to pocket size and will fit two people
- Plastic sheeting
- Pencils and paper
- Needles and thread
- Pliers
- Duct tape
- Face masks or dense-weave cotton material for nose and mouth protection
- Aluminum foil
- Plastic storage containers
- Flares
- A wrench
- A map of the area
- Toilet paper, paper towels, individually wrapped moist towelettes, feminine supplies and personal-hygiene items
- Plastic garbage bags for personal-sanitation disposal
- A plastic bucket with a tight lid
- Soap
- Liquid detergent
- Disinfectant and household chlorine bleach

- Diapers and bottles
- Any hygiene products required by older adults
- Denture needs
- Contact lenses and supplies or spare eyeglasses
- At least one complete change of clothing and footwear for each family member, including sturdy, comfortable shoes or work boots, rain gear, warm clothing, and thermal underwear
- Blankets or sleeping bags
- Hats, gloves, and sunglasses

 Essential

During a biological terrorist attack, germs may be released, causing illness if inhaled or absorbed through cuts. That's why it's important to pack and store facemasks or densely woven cotton fabric to cover your nose and mouth and designed to fit all members of the family, including your children.

Some disasters cause pieces of tiny microscopic debris to fill the air; flooding may create airborne mold causing illness and explosions may release very fine particles that can cause lung damage. Make sure to pack some heavyweight plastic garbage bags, plastic sheeting, duct tape, and scissors so that you can improvise for various situations to protect your nose, mouth, eyes, and cuts in your skin.

Be careful to store wills, Social Security cards, immunization records, insurance policies, stocks and bonds, contracts, deeds, passports, and bank and credit-card account numbers in a portable, waterproof container or airtight plastic bag. Include an inventory of valuable household goods, important telephone numbers, and family records such as birth, marriage, and death certificates.

Change and replace your stored water, food, and battery supply every six months, and evaluate your kit and your family needs at least once a year. Your doctor or pharmacist can advise you about obtaining and storing prescription medications.

Situations You May Encounter

Weather emergencies like hurricanes, tornadoes, and earthquakes may be some of the more common disaster situations you encounter. Remember, though there are some areas of the country where certain disasters are more likely to strike (for example, tornadoes in the states that encompass "Tornado Alley"), most states and territories in every region of the country have a moderate to high risk. No matter where you live or what you may need to be prepared for, it's essential to plan and prepare to weather any storm and to know what to do if told to evacuate. In addition to weather disasters, there are a variety of other emergency situations you may be faced with, including chemical, biological, or terrorist attacks.

Biological Attacks

A biological attack is the release of germs or other organic substances in a deliberate attempt to make people sick. In case of a biological attack, you will need to rely on public-health officials to provide information on how to act. During the time it takes them to determine the illness, who and how to treat, and who is in danger, continue to watch TV, listen to the radio, and check the Internet for updates. You need to know if you are among the group authorities consider infected, what signs and symptoms to be aware of, if there are medicines or vaccines available and how they are distributed, who the medicine is available to, and where to go to get emergency medical care if you develop symptoms. As always, use common sense, good hygiene and cleanliness measures, and seek medical advice.

 Fact

During a time of biological attack, if you become sick be concerned, but don't assume you need emergency-room treatment or that you are ill due to the biological attack. Your illness may just be a garden-variety sickness that happens to crop up at the same time as the attack.

Modes of entry with biological agents may vary; some must be inhaled, enter through the skin, or be ingested in order to make you sick. Some biological agents are contagious, like the smallpox virus, and some are not, such as anthrax. A biological attack may or may not be an obvious event like an explosion or a fire, but there may be subtle signs like a group of employees reporting similar illnesses and all seeking emergency care during the same time frame.

You are apt to learn of imminent threat from a TV broadcast, an emergency radio, or other signal. Any time you are alerted to a suspicious release of an unknown substance nearby, attempt to get away as quickly as possible. Cover your mouth and nose with as many layers of cloth as you can that will still allow you to breathe, such as layers of a T-shirt, towel, paper towel, or handkerchief, Wash immediately with soap and water, and contact your local authorities.

Chemical Attacks

A chemical attack is the release of a toxic gas, liquid, or solid in a deliberate attempt to poison people and the environment. Signs of a chemical attack are watery eyes, twitching, choking, breathing difficulties, and loss of coordination in all the people around you, along with signs of a poisoned atmosphere such as seeing many sick or dead small animals, birds, or fish.

When you see these signs of a chemical attack, try to identify where the chemical is coming from and the area affected, and immediately leave the area. If you are in a contaminated building, attempt to leave while avoiding the contaminated area, or stay inside the building, move as far away from the chemical release as possible, and seal the room. If you are outside, use the fastest way to get away from the chemical threat, or consider whether it would be safer to go inside a building and secure a shelter-in-place.

If you are having symptoms, immediately strip and wash with a hose, fountain, shower, or any other available source of water. Use soap if available, but don't scrub the chemical into your skin. Seek emergency medical attention as quickly as possible.

Nuclear Attacks

A nuclear blast is an explosion of widespread radioactive material involving intense light and heat, and an intense destructive pressure wave that contaminates the ground, air, and water for miles. In the case of an enormous fireball and intense flash, immediately take cover below ground if you can, or use any shield or shelter to help protect you from the pressure wave and immediate effects of the blast. A thick shield between your body, the blast, and the wave will help to absorb more of the radiation. Distance from the explosion and the amount of time you are exposed also decrease your degree of radiation exposure.

Dirty Bombs

A radiation threat known as a dirty bomb is the use of ordinary explosives in order to spread radioactive materials over a planned area of attack. It is not a nuclear explosion; the force of the blast and the radioactive contamination are more localized. In a dirty-bomb explosion, the blast is obvious, but the presence of radiation cannot be detected without the use of trained personnel and specialized equipment. Because there is radiation present, you need to take the same steps to limit your exposure: shielding, distance, and time.

Terrorism

The nature of terrorism implies that there may be little or no warning, so you need to stay alert and be aware of your surroundings when you travel, as well as in daily life including:

- Always be concerned and aware of any unusual or noticeably alarming behavior.
- Don't ever accept packages from strangers or leave luggage unattended.
- When you are staying in hotels or when you frequent certain buildings, learn where emergency exits are located.
- Notice and be cautious of objects that are heavy or breakable that could move, fall, or shatter in an explosion.
- Create a plan in response to a terrorist attack for specific features of your life and work, including such concerns as living and working in high-rise buildings.

You can deal with a terrorist incident using many of the same techniques used to prepare for other emergencies and crises. Because your family may not be together when disaster strikes, it is important to create a comprehensive advanced plan together for any scenario you might encounter, so that you all remain safe.

Resources

These resources are designed to give you more first-aid information, including where to find first-aid and basic life-support training, because it's important to have actual training and experience along with this manual. You can also visit some of the recommended Web sites and other resources for any questions you may have. For problems where you may need professional help, support, or even crisis intervention, there's a list of crisis hotlines and support organizations for you to access.

There is a wealth of information available through various Web sites to help you put together the information you need, such as prepared emergency-contact forms and checklists to help you create your disaster plan and supplies list. There are also many sites and organizations available to add to your knowledge base of first aid, injury and illness prevention, preparedness, addiction problems, mental health, and overall health care, including diet and exercise.

Web sites

The American Heart Association
www.americanheart.org
Offers an abundance of health information and comprehensive training resources for first aid and basic life support (CPR); even offers such things as recipes and cookbooks.

The American Red Cross
www.redcross.org

A place to find up-to-date information on first-aid classes, basic life support and other training, community services, disaster preparedness, blood donation, jobs, and more.

Medline Plus
www.nlm.nih.gov/medlineplus/firstaid.html

A comprehensive source for first aid, covering most injuries and illnesses.

MedicineNet.com
www.medicinenet.com/first_aid/index.htm

A comprehensive source for first aid that also includes other topics such as diet, exercise, medications, and nutrition.

Med Help
www.med-help.net/First-Aid.htm

Although it includes first aid, you can also go beyond first aid at this site and learn such things as taking blood pressure and listening to heart sounds.

Federal Emergency Management Agency
www.fema.gov

Agency to protect the nation from all hazards, including natural disasters, acts of terrorism, and other man-made disasters with a comprehensive emergency-management system of preparedness, protection, response, recovery, and mitigation.

Ready.gov
www.ready.gov
1-800-BE-READY

A site to educate and empower Americans to prepare for emergencies, including natural disasters and potential terrorist attacks, with comprehensive planning including easy-to-fill-out forms and checklists.

Occupational Safety & Health Administration
www.osha.gov
Offers safety-training videos, DVDs, software, and booklets, a complete line of safety and labor-law posters, equipment, first-aid kits, and more for your workplace health and safety, as well as first aid and disaster preparedness.

FireSafety.gov
www.firesafety.gov
This site is an information resource for eliminating residential fire deaths.

EMSResponder.com
www.emsresponder.com
A site that provides information and resources for the emergency medical-service responder, and offers a platform for online discussion and interaction.

The National Association of Free Clinics
www.freeclinics.us
A nonprofit site that provides advocacy and services to free clinics throughout the United States.

The National Library of Medicine
www.nlm.nih.gov
The world's largest medical library for research and medical information of all kinds, including finding a doctor.

National Alliance on Mental Illness
www.nami.org
A site offering advocacy, research, support, and education for persons living with serious mental illness and their families.

Kristin Brooks Hope Center

www.hopeline.com

A site whose mission is preventing suicide and educating people about depressive disorders.

The National Suicide Prevention Lifeline

www.suicidepreventionlifeline.org

A twenty-four-hour, toll-free suicide-prevention service that is available to anyone in crisis.

Planned Parenthood

www.plannedparenthood.org

This well-known organization provides information on teen pregnancy and birth control, and information related to sexual health to people of any age group.

Testicular Self-Exam (TSE)

www.adam.about.com/encyclopedia/Testicular-self-examination.htm

An overall guide to the early detection of testicular cancer by self-examination of testicles.

Sexual Violence Prevention

www.cdc.gov/ncipc/dvp/SVPrevention.htm

Information related to prevention of sexual violence.

Steroid Abuse

www.steroidabuse.org

Information about the health dangers of steroid abuse for parents and teens.

The National Youth Violence Prevention Resource Center

www.safeyouth.org

This site has information to keep your children safe, and also has sections especially for teens, health providers, and more. Topics include bullying, depression, and teen violence.

Overeaters Anonymous

www.oa.org

A place to connect with support groups, and basic information on finding the support you need on all issues regarding overeating.

The National Association for Anorexia Nervosa and Associated Eating Disorders

www.anad.org

Comprehensive information on eating disorders and where to find help.

National Domestic Violence Hotline

www.ndvh.org

Information on the prevention of domestic violence, and help for those in situations of violence and abuse.

Alcoholics Anonymous World Services, Inc.

www.aa.org

The primary purpose of AA is to stay sober and to support others with the same goal. AA provides a recovery process and support network in chapters worldwide.

About Alcoholism and Drug Abuse

www.alcoholism.about.com

This site has information covering alcohol and substance abuse, including such things as self-assessment tests so that you can better understand and come to grips with your need for help and intervention.

National Clearing House for Alcohol and Drug Information

www.ncadi.samhsa.gov

A comprehensive resource regarding substance and alcohol abuse for you and your teen.

Al-Anon and Alateen

www.al-anon.org

A site providing information and support for teens and families affected by alcohol abuse.

Narcotics Anonymous World Services, Inc.

www.na.org

Narcotics Anonymous is an international association comprised of recovering drug addicts that provides a recovery process and support network in chapters worldwide.

American Council for Drug Education

www.acde.org

An information resource for drugs and drug-abuse education.

National HIV Testing Resources

www.hivtest.org

A comprehensive national information resource for AIDS/HIV education.

Smoking Cessation at About.com

www.quitsmoking.about.com

This site has comprehensive information on how to quit smoking, with statistics about smoking, tips for prevention, and other great information to help you quit.

National Center for Missing and Exploited Children

www.missingkids.com

You will find incredible and comprehensive information at this site on how to talk to children about staying safe.

Hotlines

The National Suicide Prevention Lifeline

1-800-273-TALK (1-800-273-8255)

The National Suicide Prevention Lifeline is a toll-free suicide hotline with information on suicide for families and support lines for anyone in crisis.

National Domestic Violence Hotline
1-800-799-SAFE (7233), 1-800-787-3224(TTY)
Support and advocacy for those in abusive relationships.

Cocaine Hotline
1-800-COCAINE
Information and resources regarding cocaine abuse.

NIDA Hotline
1-800-622-HELP
Referral service for cocaine users.

National Suicide Hotline
1-800-SUICIDE
A support line to help during crises, prevent suicide, and educate people about all depressive disorders.

National Youth Violence Prevention Resource Center
NYVPRC@safeyouth.org
1-866-SAFEYOUTH (1-866-723-3968), 1-866-620-4160 (TTY)
A support line to help stop youth violence before it starts.

National Child Abuse Hotline
1-800-4-A-CHILD (1-800-422-4453)
A site to get help for issues of child abuse and neglect.

National Sexual Assault Hotline
1-800-656-HOPE (1-800-656-4673)
A support line to help stop youth sexual violence before it starts.

National Hopeline Network
1-800-SUICIDE (1-800-784-2433)
A suicide-prevention hotline giving help and support during crises.

National Mental Health Association
1-800-969-NMHA
A help line for any mental-health problem or issue.

American Academy of Child and Adolescent Psychiatry
1-202-966-7300
A line for referrals to psychiatrists who work with children and teens.

Suicide Prevention Action Network USA
1-202- 499-3600
Will give referrals for support, treatment, and help for any mental-health crisis.

Organizations

The American Heart Association
www.americanheart.org
1-800-AHA-USA-1 or 1-800-242-8721, ASA: 1-888-4-STROKE or 1-888-478-7653, AHA Professional Membership: 1-800-787-8984 or Outside U.S.: 1-301-223-2307
Offers an abundance of health information and comprehensive training resources for first aid and basic life support (CPR); even offers such things as recipes and cookbooks.

The American Red Cross
www.redcross.org
A place to find up-to-date information on first-aid classes, basic life support, and other training, community services, disaster preparedness, blood donation, jobs, and more.

Centers for Disease Control

www.cdc.gov

Government site for anything you need to know about international travel and overall health.

PandemicFlu.gov

www.pandemicflu.gov

Comprehensive government site to prepare the public for pandemic flu.

Ready.gov

www.ready.gov

Comprehsive government site to prepare the public for any type of disaster.

Medic First Aid International

www.medicfirstaid.us

1-800-800-7099

A worldwide leader in CPR/first-aid emergency-care training programs for business, industry, and the public.

Boy Scouts of America

www.scouting.org

Prepares young men to make ethical and moral choices over their lifetimes, and includes programs to teach boys first aid.

Girl Scouts of the USA

www.girlscouts.org

1-800-GSUSA 4 U[1-8001478-7248]or 1-212-852-8000

Prepares girls by building character and skills for success in the real world, and has programs including those to teach girls first aid.

Alcoholics Anonymous World Services, Inc.

www.aa.org

1-212-870-3400

The primary purpose of AA is to stay sober and to support others with the same goal.

American Academy of Pediatrics (AAP)
www.aap.org
Learn about your pediatrician, check references, and learn about current policy.

American Academy of Child and Adolescent Psychiatry
www.aacap.org
1-202-966-7300
Help understanding childhood mental illness, including facts you need to know and where to find help in your area.

American Psychological Association
1-800-964-2000
www.helping.apa.org
Find a psychologist and learn more about how they can treat mental-health problems.

National Council on Alcoholism Information
1-800-NAC-CALL
A referral service for anyone seeking help for substance and alcohol abuse.

Books

American Heart Association. *Fitting in Fitness: Hundreds of Simple Ways to Put More Physical Activity into Your Life.* (Clarkson Potter; reissue edition, 1997)

Karen Buhler Gale, Karen Buhler, David Buchholz. *The Kids' Guide to First Aid: All about Bruises, Burns, Stings, Sprains & Other Ouches.* (Vanwell Publishing Ltd., 2002)

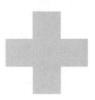

Additional Safety Tips

When summer comes, it's easy to let your guard down when all you want to do is have fun on your vacations and time off, going to the pool and the beach, or to the mountains for hiking and camping. But even with all your fun activities, you have to keep your health and safety in mind no matter the season or the holiday.

Water Safety

The best way to stay safe around water is to know how to swim, so if you or your children don't already know how to swim, take lessons at the local public pool or the American Red Cross. Make sure to always swim with a friend; accidents in the water are frequent and the water is one place you should never be alone. When swimming at the beach or local water hole, make sure to only swim in supervised areas and to obey all rules and posted signs. Also, if you know that the weather conditions are going to be bad, you should not go swimming, or should stop and get out of the water if there is any indication that bad weather is coming.

Never drink alcohol and swim—just as with driving, alcohol impairs your judgment, balance, and coordination while it lessens your body's ability to stay warm in the water. So drinking while swimming is going to affect your swimming and diving skills, and make it more likely for you to be injured or have a near-drowning incident.

Bicycling

Biking is fun at any age, but requires some planning and prevention because bike accidents are too common.

- Wear protective clothing including helmets to prevent significant injuries, including fatal head injuries.
- Reflective clothing is a must for nighttime or low-visibility conditions, along with bicycle-safety equipment such as reflectors on the frame and wheels.
- Ride the right bike for the right conditions; if you are off-roading you should be riding a mountain bike.
- Maintain your bikes so that everything works, including the brakes, and there will be less chance of getting flats that could cause you to fall and be injured.
- Practice and be confident before riding in traffic and on public roads, use correct hand signals when turning, and always ride following the rules of the road.
- Ride at the proper speed, yield the right of way, and don't ride while or after drinking alcohol.
- Be aware of car doors opening; uneven surfaces, such things as sewer covers, debris on roads; and poorly lit areas.
- Ride in single file along with traffic, not against it, and don't ride on major roads or on sidewalks.

- When you are going to pass someone on bike or walking trails, announce yourself by yelling out, "On your left."

Take a little care before and while you are biking so that you and your family can enjoy riding together safely. Always supervise young children, and only let them ride in enclosed areas.

Halloween Safety

Halloween is a time-honored tradition, but also one that brings a lot of excitement and sometimes lack of carefulness. Most Halloween accidents happen from falls and pedestrian-versus-car crashes. A little foresight can make this night much safer for everyone. Motorists need to take special care to be alert on Halloween and to watch for children who may be darting out from between cars and running across streets. Children may be in places you least expect them, such as walking on roadways, medians, and jumping off curbs, so you need to take care when exiting and entering driveways, roads, and alleys. Keep an eye out for children in dark clothing the entire evening. Some other Halloween tips include:

- All children under age twelve need to have an adult or an older, responsible youth supervising them while they go door to door.
- Give children a route to follow and instruct them not to go anywhere else, to only stop at houses or apartment

buildings that are well lit, and to never go into a stranger's home.

- Have set times for children to be out and to be home.
- Go over all your trick-or-treat safety rules and precautions, including safety rules for walking on the road and curbs.
- Pin an identification paper on all children with their name, address, and phone number in case anyone gets lost or separated from the group.
- Use fire-retardant materials for costumes and have them loose enough for the kids to wear warm clothes underneath.
- To prevent falls, make sure the costumes aren't too long or that there is anything else that could be a tripping hazard.
- Make costumes with a light-colored fabric, and reinforce the costumes and the bags children carry with reflective tape to make the children visible.
- Instead of masks that obscure your child's vision, use makeup, but make sure the ingredients state, "Made with U.S.-Approved Color Additives," "Laboratory Tested," "Meets Federal Standards for Cosmetics," or "Nontoxic," and follow the package instructions for application.
- Make sure any masks have nose, mouth, and eye holes large enough to really see and breathe through.
- Don't ever let children carry sharp objects; make things like knives and swords from cardboard or other flexible materials.

- Give the kids flashlights to carry so they can see better, and also so they can be more easily seen by motorists.

Instruct your kids to walk, not run, from house to house; to not run across yards and lawns where they might trip on unseen hazards; to walk on sidewalks, never in the street; and to walk facing traffic if there are no sidewalks on the left side of the road. Finally, make sure your kids show you their treats before they eat anything, and if you have any doubts about a treat, throw it out.

Holiday-Season Safety

It's the most wonderful time of the year—to gather with friends and family, to eat lots of good food, to decorate, and to exchange presents and good will. But it's also a time to be very conscious of any potential holiday health and safety hazards such as depression, accidents, allergies, and alcohol-related problems so that you can have a truly enjoyable and joyful holiday season.

Holiday Heartburn

The holidays are synonymous with food, and even binging for some. Eating too much can cause you to gain weight, and it can also lead to heartburn and a condition called gastroesophageal reflux disease (GERD), which is acid backing up into the esophagus. If you already suffer from GERD, then holidays are going to be an additional challenge for you. The best treatment for heartburn is to not overeat and drink plenty of nonalcoholic and non-caffeinated fluids throughout the day. Avoid eating white foods like refined sugar, potatoes, and white rice; refined, processed foods; and fried foods; and drinking coffee and alcohol. Try to space out your meals and make them smaller and more frequent. If you have nighttime symptoms, try elevating the head of your bed four to six inches and eat your last meal two to four hours before bedtime.

Holiday Allergies

People who have asthma and allergies have added health challenges during the holidays. It's a good idea to be especially careful of any known triggers and to take your medications as prescribed. In order to avoid any problems with food allergies, make sure to ask your guests if they have any allergies so that you can prepare a safe feast without any of the ingredients that will cause someone to be ill or have an allergic reaction. If you have been prescribed an epinephrine injection kit, take it with you when you eat out and make sure others are aware that it's available in case of a reaction.

Environmental Allergies

To prepare for the changing seasons and the allergies they aggravate when you are working outside, try to remove any wet dirt and leaves from your house foundation and gutters, and stack all firewood outside—only bring new logs in for immediate use. To avoid winter allergens, also wear gloves and a facemask when doing outdoor chores. Inside the house, dust and clean off decorations and ornaments, replace or clean furnace filters, and avoid scented candles, potpourri, and other scented items that can cause discomfort for those with sensitivities. Dust and scents may be irritants even to those without allergies. If you know you have severe sensitivities to dust, there are special facemasks you can buy to wear while you are cleaning out your winter decorations. Avoid buying mountain-cedar Christmas trees because they are the most allergenic, and be very cautious if using spray-on snow or pine-scented sprays or oils because they can all cause allergic reactions. Also be sure to keep your tree watered so that mold will not grow.

Holiday Drinking

The holidays typically involve alcohol, with myriad office parties and social events and family get-togethers. As during the rest of the year, moderation is the key. Most people who overindulge have had the unfortunate experience of too much alcohol, causing overeating, sometimes promiscuity, impairment to driving, and much more. It's also very high in calories and only adds to the holiday weight problems, and too many drinks at one time, as can happen at some parties, causes alcohol poisoning. Pregnant women and women trying to get pregnant should not drink, as alcohol during pregnancy has serious consequences on the growth and development of the fetus, a condition known as fetal alcohol syndrome. Anyone with a history of alcoholism or alcohol abuse has even more temptations with alcohol at parties, feasts, and get-togethers.

If you know someone who has a problem or difficulty saying no to alcohol, help them out by making it unavailable when they are visiting. And when you are going out, give yourself a limit so that you don't become a statistic, designate a driver, and stop yourself from doing anything you might regret.

Holiday Decoration Safety

Holiday decorations are a fixture of the winter holidays, but when they are not used properly, they can result in fires, injuries, and even fatalities. According to the U.S. Consumer Product Safety Commission, about 12,500 people every year are treated in emergency departments from falls, cuts, shocks, and burns caused by dried-out Christmas trees, broken or faulty holiday lights, and other decorations. There are about 300 fires a year leading to 10 deaths involving Christmas trees, including about $10 million in property damage and loss.

- Artificial trees should be labeled, "Fire Resistant."
- Live trees need to be fresh, with green needles that are firmly on and not dry (test your tree by tapping it on the ground; it's fresh if most of the needles stay on the tree).
- Never set up your tree near a fireplace, radiator, doorway, or any other traffic area, and keep the tree stand filled with water.
- All lights should have labels stating that they were tested for safety by a recognized laboratory like the UL (Underwriters Laboratories).

- Don't use broken lights, lights with cracked sockets, frayed or bare wires, or loose connections.
- Don't leave lights on when you go to bed or leave the house.
- Only use noncombustible or flame-retardant materials for tree trimming, and never use lighted candles on a tree.
- Keep all sharp and breakable decorations away from children, as well as any small, removable parts, decorations, and toys.
- Always keep a screen on your fireplace to prevent any sparks from igniting nearby flammable Christmas decorations.

Holiday Stress

Probably the biggest mental-health issues around the holidays are stress, fatigue, and anxiety. Holidays often cause self-reflection and loneliness because they cause people to think of the past or of loved ones who aren't there or who have died. In order to keep low moods at bay, keep your routine as stable as you can, exercise and eat right, and limit alcohol. You may find that you actually enjoy yourself more if you don't overindulge with food and drink, if you do get enough sleep, and pace yourself. To make sure you do this, plan ahead of time and set limits for yourself for when you need to stop drinking or eating. Also remember that you have personal physical, emotional, and financial limitations and you can't be everything to everyone or give what you don't have. Remember to look at the holidays as a new beginning with opportunities for the future instead of regrets about the past, and this includes setting realistic New Year's resolutions. Be careful and stay safe during the holidays so you can have a truly joyous season.

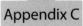

Emergency Contacts

Poison Control Center

Ambulance

Fire Department

Police Department

Hospital Emergency Department

Doctor's Name

Doctor's Phone Number

Health-Insurance Plan

Health-Insurance Policy Number

Emergency-Contact Name

Emergency-Contact Phone Number

Relationship

Mom's Work   Mom's Cell

Dad's Work   Dad's Cell

Full Name

Date of Birth

Allergies

Medical Conditions

Blood Type

Index